Gene Ladd

Amber Waves of Gain

How the Government Makes Us Fat, and the Spiritual Power to Lose It

Published by Pleasant Stone Farm, Ltd.

For discounted quantity orders for this book, contact the author at geneladd@usa.net

DEDICATION

This book is dedicated to all the people I have seen who walk with their eyes downcast because they are not comfortable with the way they appear and feel in their own body. May they gain control and find the image and joy God intends for their lives...

CONTENTS

VERY IMPORTANT

We are created with unique qualities and gifts. No single set of guidelines can be right for all of us without some modifications to make them work in our best interest. Before beginning a major change in diet or lifestyle always discuss your plans with your doctor or healthcare professional.

INTRODUCTION

Obesity in America is not the illness; it is one of several symptoms of a deep, pervasive sickness that infects our whole political process. It is greed and it has corrupted our regulatory agencies. The agencies of government that are tax funded to protect us through regulation of agriculture, medicine and other staples of life have become the benefactors of those they allege to regulate. Profits and dollars are the measure of value. Nutrition and health are not as important as the commerce that surrounds them. Our food supply system is producing nearly double the amount of calories that the average person needs per day, and the U.S. Department of Agriculture is prompting us to consume them. The USDA mission is a thriving agricultural economy, even if it is achieved at the expense of the health and wellbeing of the people who are taxed for its protection. As a result of these political and distorted conditions we have become overfed and under-nourished.

The symptoms of this corrupt gluttony only begin with obesity. There is a condition that has come to be called Syndrome X and according to the American Medical Association it can lead to heart disease, diabetes, arthritis, many forms of cancer and other totally preventable illnesses. Washington is obsessed with doing something about the cost of healthcare. Our nation is divided over the Affordable Care Act. Meanwhile it only addresses ways to pay for the ever rising costs of healthcare. It so far fails to address ways to reduce the burden of care the system has thrust upon the medical community. The care givers are overwhelmed by the case load of food related and preventable diseases. Our treasury is threatened as healthcare takes larger and larger chunks of our Gross National Product each year: 2.6 Trillion in 2010, up from 256 Billion in 1980. A recent estimate from the Surgeon General indicated that 75% of all visits to doctors were for diet related conditions. More recent estimates indicate that perhaps as many as 90% of the people being treated by the healthcare system today would not need to be seen by a doctor if they consumed a proper diet.

The average American diet today is filled with empty calories and a host of toxins that disrupt the workings of the body rather than nourish it. In some cases the basic food is compromised. In others, there are approved additives that challenge the body of those who consume them: monosodium glutamate, aspartame and other artificial sweeteners, and the natural sweeteners such as High Fructose Corn Syrup and Fructose Concentrate. Sugar gets the blame, but few products actually contain old fashioned sugar. In fact, sugar has become a desirable ingredient to be found in healthier products. Then there is a growing list of pesticides and herbicides used on the farm that leave residues in and on the products. Procedures such as irradiation and microwaving change the molecular structure of the food. Toxins such as Bisphenol A are created from the packaging. All things considered, the human body is pretty amazing to survive the punishment we give it.

All we hear from our leaders is that we have become too sedentary with our computers and smart phones. "Get more exercise", we are told. I am tired of being told that I am lazy and not motivated. At which end of my twelve-hour day would you have me pop into the gym? The bureaucratic mindset holds the belief that we Americans are glutinously greedy and indulgent, and that we are too lazy to "work it off." Actually *greed* and *gluttony* are involved here, but in places other than our dinner tables and lunch counters. The damaging greed and gluttony can be found prevailing around the conference tables in corporate board rooms where determinations are made concerning how to get government subsidies or bend the regulations to accommodate the use of more toxins.

This condition is facilitated by an easily documented bureaucratic reality known as the ***Revolving Door***. Most appointees to positions at the FDA, USDA and EPA are recruited from firms regulated by the agency. When they leave these agencies they have usually earned themselves a choice position with the firms they regulated, or at a company owned by a regulated firm. It is a tight world and the power brokers know who their friends are and remember them with appropriate rewards. There will be stories told in the chapters ahead that demonstrate the effect the **Revolving Door** has on our health and the epidemic of obesity.

We have grown accustomed to stories of abuse in procurement at the Pentagon: thousand dollar ash trays and even more expensive toilet seats. What most of us do not realize is that most other agencies of government operate in a similar climate of abuse. The curse of prosperity is the immeasurable amounts of money government can waste and pocket, even in recession. In the fall of 2012 our Congress has not been able to even agree on a budget for three years, but there was bipartisan support for the most corrupt Farm Bill ever drafted. It will guarantee government subsidies to families with incomes well into six figures. It will reward the politically connected a bountiful harvest of tax subsidies for not producing. Even with draught conditions, the US farm harvest this year according to the USDA will be among the best ever. As the year ended Congress could not find a way to pay for the new legislation, so the old Farm Bill was continued to Septermber 2013. That is another convenience of running what is supposed to be the strongest government on the planet without putting together a real budget. The Farm Bill was needed in WWII to stabilize prices and maintain food production. The parasites of politics soon learned they could tap the treasury by manipulating the provisions of the bill. Today the legislation is written to accommodate the parasites. The average income of those getting hand-outs from the USDA is $135,000 and their average business debt is no more than 9%. Something to think about since the government has to borrow or print the money to fund the Farm Bill. Food production would prosper in an open market. In fact, the legislation makes it more difficult for small sustainable family farms to reach the market with their harvests. They exist in a subculture of farms stands supported by astute individuals who are eager to avoid the health challenges of the mainstream food processing and delivery system.

Our subject is obesity, and I will be compelled to raise issues concerning the *genetic modification* of food crops in the U.S. and around the world now that a Norwegian study has linked genetically modified corn to weight gain. *The Environmental Working Group* estimates that Americans are eating more than their weight in genetically modified foods each year. In most cases, we may not even know that we are eating GMOs. EWG calculated that the average American annually consumes genetically engineered foods in these quantities: 68 pounds of beet sugar, 58 pounds of corn syrup, 38 pounds of soybean oil and 29 pounds of corn-based products, for a total of 193 pounds. It is estimated that the average adult in the U.S. weighs 179 pounds,

Shortly after discoveries in genetic science were announced, Monsanto executives devised a mission to control the world food supply by controlling the distribution of seeds. The company set about to genetically modify ancient strains of seeds and to record them as intellectual property. In other words they got a patent on the seed. US Courts, the World Court and Courts in other countries have sustained the patents. Farmers everywhere have been banned from saving seeds and are forced to buy new seeds each year. After the invasion of Iraq farmers were told they could not use the seeds they had saved for years. They had to buy patented seeds. That may have made explaining the benefits of the "democracy" we were introducing a bit more difficult. Monsanto holds patents on 90% of the genetically modified seeds in use today. The modifications make the seeds immune to chemical herbicides and pesticides, but at the same time increase the need for these chemicals to support their growth to harvest. In only a very few years the chemicals overwhelm the soil and it has to go fallow for several years before it can be cultivated again. This has forced Monsanto and other chemical giants to clear vast acreage of rain forest to cultivate the modified seeds. The biggest challenge to what we have come to call our carbon footprint is not the use of fossil fuel that releases carbon into the atmosphere; it is the loss of oxygen producing foliage in the rain forest that converts the carbon to fresh air.

Only a minimum amount of testing has been carried out to determine if the genetic modifications might raise health issues for those who consume the food. Many negative results have been found, but Monsanto continues to expand its mission without meaningful opposition. Monsanto, perhaps more than any other company, has used the ***Revolving Door*** to its benefit.

Aside from the harm genetic modification is doing to our food supply system and the massive corruption that supports it, I share a personal repugnance to it. Taking genes from one species and splicing them into another in a combination that would never have occurred in nature is immoral. These combinations have included: fish into tomatoes, frog into potato and dangerous bacteria such as anthrax into our dairy and beef production. The introduction of rBGH growth hormone into our dairy and beef supply remains a disgrace. This product is banned in every industrialized nation except the US, Mexico and Brazil because of its potential threat of cancer. It also carries a potential for increased body weight and such things a pernicious puberty.

Above, I said that sustainable family farms exist in a subculture. It is under serious attack. In California a swat team raided a raw food co-op and destroyed the inventory. The owner and some employees were detained. The EPA has raided small farms declaring that hay is a bio-hazard. In Tennessee Federal Agents closed down a bulk food supplier and tried to get a list of customers. The list was not given up. The agents went door to door trying to find the people who were hoarding food supplies. People have been threatened with jail and fines for growing gardens on their own property. Many of these actions were taken for violations of zoning and deed covenants, but who is to say that a lawn is more pleasing to the eye than rows of beautiful vegetables and berries. If one has more sun in the front yard than the back yard, the front yard is a better choice for a garden. There is a constant undercurrent that seems to be trying to criminalize every aspect of natural health; whether it is fresh raw food or herbs and supplements. Frankly, I do not appreciate being classified as a criminal when I drink raw milk and eat something from my garden grown from heirloom seeds.

The truth of the matter is that it is our food that makes people fat: not their genes, not a virus, not a missing chemical in the body. It is the food, not the way the Earth gave it to us, but rather the way it is manipulated for longer shelf life and higher profits. Profits are not sinful. Profits are the fruits of labor. But when profits are made without labor at the expense of those who have paid good money to people who are entrusted to make sure their food is safe and nutritious, it is a shameful corruption that has a deadly outcome. We can no longer afford to be healthy. We do not have and cannot make enough money to be healthy within the current system. Healthcare will continue to cost more than we can afford for a quality of life that we cannot long endure. The only answer is not within our political capabilities. The only answer will come from cooperating with the *Laws of Nature* and the Earth.

∽∽

Obesity and Fat Cats

I am tired of being told that I need to get more exercise. I take care of sixteen acres and cut wood for the winter. Everybody I know is going to a gym or walking and cycling. The bureaucratic mindset holds a belief that we Americans are glutinously greedy and indulgent, and that we are too lazy to "work it off." Greed and gluttony are involved, but in higher places that our homes. The real greed and the true cause of our national obesity are found at the conference tables in some corporate board rooms. Obesity in America is nothing more than one of the symptoms of a sickness that has seized control of our political system. The very government regulatory agencies that are supposed to guard our health and wellbeing are telling us to eat the adulterated food that is abundant, not the foods we need. A surplus of some food items, such as wheat and corn, is created by tax supported subsidies. These are the foods we are encouraged to consume, because they are plentiful, not because they are good for us or good for the Earth. The USDA, Department of Agriculture wants us to get half our calories from grains. We actually produce nearly twice the calories needed per person, and we are urged to consume them because it is good for the economy. Nutrition is never a consideration in the production of these government manipulated foods.

If you are like me you are tired of being told that the only way to control your weight is to get more exercise. It appears that every official of government at every level of public health and authority wants to blame obesity on human weakness and laziness. We are weak and lazy when it comes to deciding who will serve us in public office. When it comes to health and weight control, we are trying to find the truth. We are not an obese nation because we use our cars and spend time with our TVs and Smart Phones. The only answer they have for obesity is exercise. The truth is the official U.S. public health sector, the regulatory agencies such as the FDA and USDA, designated to guard our quality of life and health is responsible for approving the conditions that are causing the epidemic of obesity.

Over time, public health recommendations have come to represent the goals of the food producers and vendors, rather than the health needs of the American public. Policy is shaped by political influence exerted by trade associations and lobbyists who represent factory farming, food distributors, grocery stores, restaurants and every other sector of the food delivery and supply chain. It is this corruption and distortion of the food delivery system that is causing ill health and particularly obesity. Greedy and powerful corporate interests can get public health officials to support any agenda that supports profits. If we become ill from the food, we begin to support another greed-driven sector, healthcare. So goes the vicious cycle and the health and quality of life of the average American citizen are eroded daily. What is the answer? Drop out. Stop believing the lies and deceptions. You must take control of your life at every level, especially food and beverage choices.

A few years ago the seriousness of the situation was underscored by an article in *The New England Journal of Medicine* in which it predicted a drop in the life expectancy of American citizens by at least five years because of obesity and related diseases. For decades American waistlines have continued to expand despite a booming business in diets and exercise programs. Not only are more of us reaching the point of obesity, but also it is happening at younger and younger ages. Young people are experiencing conditions of diabetes and heart disease more commonly than ever before. Teenagers are found to have the clogged veins found usually in a person in their 40s or 50s. So many young people are developing diabetes that the name of the disease has been changed. It was once called ***adult onset diabetes*** because people developed in when they were mature adults, normally mid-life. More than half the cases of diabetes are among people under 20 years of age. Thus the name change from ***Adult Onset Diabetes*** to ***Type Two Diabetes***. Recent government figures show that at least two thirds of the population is overweight with actual obesity getting very close to fifty percent. We have a new classification of patient, Syndrome X: excess weight (especially around the girth), high blood pressure, insulin resistance, high blood lipids, high cholesterol and other markers for heart disease. Obesity also has strong links to cancer, arthritis and gastric or colic disorders. Obesity is tied to so many serious disorders that the *NEJM* lowered the life expectancy by at least five years. It is a haunting question: "Why is a nation obsessed with diet and exercise defiantly growing obese?" Seems as though we want to blame everything but the food we eat. As I will discuss later, it is the food, but stress can be a factor.

Are You Stressed Out?

Some research points to growing stress as the reason for an increasingly obese population. I think stress is an easy whipping post that gets blamed for far more than it deserves. Stress is a spiritual issue. We tend to, as the saying goes, "Sweat the small stuff, and avoid the important stuff." Stress is created when a system or organ of the body is asked to deliver more than it is prepared to deliver. The preparation could be deficient because of inadequate amounts of rest, fresh air, pure water, or any of the essential nutrients. Still, in some ways, stress can lead to overeating. Stress triggers secretions of added cortisol. This hormone triggers metabolism without true hunger. The metabolism causes the production of extra glucose that turns to fat, especially around the girth. How many people do you know who have normal weight in their legs and upper body, but they have a big spare tire and "love handles" over their belt? In this regard stress does cause added weight gain, but it is far from the only or even primary cause of obesity.

Many times stress is simply a lack of energy. In the work place or other social environments we are often surrounded by people who seem to emanate unhappiness. We might feel like we are in a strange land among these people as they feed on every negative viewpoint and constantly review negative events. If we are not careful, part of our protection from this situation can be weight gain. If we are open to these conversations, they can pull the energy right out of us. We can turn to quick and available snacks seeking to energize ourselves to finish the work day. If we are not careful, we might pack on a few layers of protective insulation between us and their negativity.

Among the more common and untreated stress-related conditions affecting Americans is latent acidosis. As acid levels grow higher in our bodies, oxygen is reduced and a disease-prone environment develops. Acidosis is also linked to our high-acid diets. It can mimic or lead to any number of serious diseases. There is no pill or medication to relieve the pressures of stress from our daily lives. There are some pills that might make us oblivious to this kind of stress, but they do not remove the actual stress. They only change our perceptions of it, and will most likely cause physical stress to the body with side effects, such as slower metabolism.

However, if we start the day in our peaceful garden of thought and remain there throughout the day, we have a protective shell that protects our personal space and state of being. Deep breathing, prayer and meditation, and essential nutrition are the most powerful stress busters we have.

If you want to witness a prime example of how stress leads to weight gain become a people watcher the next time you visit an automobile agency. Here is a community of people who thrive on stress and competition. They also subsist on junk food deliveries for lunch and snacks from the vending machines. You will see a 20 oz soda on most desks or in most hands. That diet will pack on the pounds without the stress, but the combination creates some embarrassing waddles for those who have been in this environment for more than a year. Sadly, you can have a similar people watching experience at a hospital or health facility. They all walk around with a 20 oz soda. If they are stressed it frequently does not show in the pace.

Emotions are another challenge. I have worked with several young women who were sexually abused as young girls. They became seriously obese for a combination of reasons not the least of which was to become unattractive and protected from the danger of unwanted advances. I had a very difficult case with a woman I can call Alice. She was a pretty young girl when she married her husband. They lived in his mother's house. Everything was fine for several months and they were very happy. Alice became pregnant and they were looking forward to starting a family. When Alice had her sonogram there was more news. She was carrying twins. A couple of days later when Alice came home from work the doors were locked and the husband and his mother would not let her in the house. They had packed her belongings and told her that there was no room in the house or their life for twins. Alice was forced to move in with her mother. As the weeks progressed she became very heavy, and after the birth of the twins she continued to gain weight. When I met her she was seriously obese and a nervous wreck. She could not come to our meetings without bringing soda and a snack. She did however learn the ropes of the public assistance available to women in her situation. Her twin girls were in college and doing well. She came to me because their graduation was a few months away and she wanted to attend without embarrassing her girls. When she realized why she was a slave to food and began to see that she was an accomplished person with many accomplishments to be proud of, she began to change her diet and her belief system. She enrolled in a swimming program and did laps every day. She lost weight and was able to walk with pride when the graduation took place.

Many people turn to food for comfort and protection. If they are consuming the food from the mainstream supply system, obesity is all but guaranteed. Everybody is different and everybody must find their own pathway to change, but all will need to change their diet to find the image of themselves they seek.

⮑⮑

Healthcare Is Sick and Overwhelmed

So far health care has not been able to stop the obesity epidemic. In many ways, healthcare itself has become a major cause of death and injury. And, in many cases, the medications prescribed by physicians such as prednisone, other steroids and common drugs, can lead to weight gain. While our American diet can be blamed for much illness, the treatment of the illness reflects the same distortion of public policy. Many believe health care has become the leading cause of death and injury in America. The report, *Death by Medicine,* makes a strong case for the belief that iatrogenesis—reactions caused by drugs, operations, and invasive procedures—is at least equal to heart disease and cancer as a leading cause of death. The first rule of healthcare is to cause no harm. When treatments bring harm, they are iatrogenic. I use this information not to criticize the dedicated people who have devoted their lives to caring for others in the medical profession, but instead to point out to readers that the figures on iatrogenic incidents do offer an important critique of our current healthcare system, despite the honest efforts of those dedicated individuals.

In fact, I believe we are experiencing a national health crisis that has overwhelmed the healthcare system. The vast majority of visits to a doctor or clinic do not involve symptoms that fit a traditional diagnosis. People see several doctors, and each one can prescribe several medications. Often the prescribed drugs conflict with those ordered by one or more other doctors. As drugs have become more powerful, the side effects have also become more pronounced—and potentially deadly. We need only watch TV commercials or read a magazine advertisement to learn that the side effects of some common medications have symptoms as severe as the condition they are supposed to treat. How can we help but doubt the safety of these drugs?

In addition, we constantly learn of medications that have been withdrawn from the market after causing severe side effects, including heart attack and death. We recall thousands of automobiles because of a minor defect, but we allow medications to remain on the market knowing they cause death and injury. Only when the death toll become conspicuous do we take them off the market. Even then, most are reintroduced with new dosing instructions. Medicine, prescribed properly by the book, is killing an average of 300 Americans every day according to the American Medical Association. It is a unique complacency, to say the least.

A Nation on Drugs

At one time, pharmaceutical drugs were developed to meet the needs of people based on their specific health problems. Today, slick marketing is often used to create a condition after the drug is developed. For example, ADD never appeared in the medical literature before the development of Ritalin. Today, it is reported that at least 20% of our young people are being given Ritalin or a similar drug, perhaps Adderall. Is it a coincidence that these drugs are also a popular street drug with an effect on the mind similar to cocaine or methadone? The FDA approves drugs based on the small studies provided by the pharmaceutical manufacturers. We assume they are safe. Within months of their introduction, however, we often learn that these drugs are harming and killing people.

According to the FDA, Vioxx, as only one example, caused around 150,000 heart attacks, with more than a third of them fatal. This means that Vioxx killed more people than all our recent wars. More concern has been expressed about what happened to the stock market with its removal than for the suffering and deaths of the people who took it.

Throughout history, farming and agriculture evolved around the needs of the people of the region. Farmers developed crops that met the needs of the people based on their preferences, the climate and nutritional needs. Today we have evolved to a place where foods are grown for profit, without regard to nutrition and the needs of those who are to consume them. As factory-farm conglomerates replaced family farms, agriculture itself has become a political process.

Today a handful of associations and lobby groups representing the major food producers have the power to shape policy. The two agencies that are on our tax supported payroll to protect our interests, the FDA and USDA, are controlled by these powerful special interest groups. Most people working for either of these agencies are on loan from the corporate sector, or they are soon to be part of the corporate sector, the **Revolving Door**. Profits determine the crops that will be raised, and the protector agencies are the pawns that help create a market for the harvest.

The USDA Food Pyramid and the subsequent guidelines and recommendations give every food lobbyist one or more servings per day. We are then promoted to support every segment of the agricultural and food economy by eating far more calories than our bodies need, while we grow ill from a lack of nutrition.

⌒⌒

The Problem with the Pyramid

One recent report estimated that a person would have to eat 10,000 calories per day of the standard American diet to achieve the modest amount of nutrition of the RDA, recommended daily allowance of vitamins and minerals. The RDA is the minimal amount of nutrients needed to avoid obvious diseases such as scurvy and beriberi. The 100% of the RDA does not come close to the nutritional needs of the human body based on the findings of the government's own National Institutes of Health.

A potent multi-vitamin and mineral complex from a health food store will contain hundreds of percentage points more than the RDA. To achieve the level of a potent multi-vitamin and mineral complex, the amount of food could be as high as 50,000 calories per day. That would be many times the amount that caused obesity and related health problems in a 30-day period during the making the documentary, *"Super-Size Me."* The American diet is very high in fat-producing calories, but extremely deficient in essential nutrients.

Shining Light on the Pyramid Scheme

In the 1980s Luise Light was the leader of the USDA scientific staffers who worked on the establishment of the first Food Pyramid. She writes that the team worked very hard to come up with dietary guidelines that would guarantee balanced nutrition for anyone who followed them. She says that they even assessed the effects of dietary shortfalls

When their work came back after review by the USDA Commissioner they were completely dismayed. The Pyramid that was published had little resemblance to the one that was developed by the scientists and nutritional experts Light had supervised. The wording was changed to favor the use of processed foods. The serving sizes were greatly increased. Today, the Pyramid and subsequent guidelines continue to reflect the agenda of the food lobby at every level with virtually no concern for the actual nutritional needs of the people.

≈≈

The Growing Need for Nutrients

This need for nutrients is not a recent development. In 1936, coming out of the Dust Bowl of the Great Depression, a report was received by the United States Senate showing that the U.S. farmland was depleted of vital and essential minerals. The report concluded that the mineral content of the agricultural soil was so low that a person would not have the stomach capacity to consume enough food to provide the daily need of minerals. In the years since 1936 we have seen many developments in farming. We have learned to produce bountiful crops with the help of chemicals and more chemicals. We grow more and bigger vegetables than we did in 1936, but we have not addressed the issue of mineral depletion. Only with the recent expansion of organic farming have we seen the soil enriched with organic materials. Sustainable farming methods are among the first requirements of organic certification. It is no mystery why organically grown foods have many times more nutrition than conventional crops.

Hungry soil is only the beginning of the nutrition problem. Let's look at the lifecycle of the plants we grow for more hints. While modern farming methods can produce large and esthetically beautiful fruits and vegetables, nutrition has not improved. In the lifecycle of a plant, its first phase is size. Once it reaches full potential for size, nature is ready to fill it with nutrients. If the soil contains minerals, the plant will pull them from the soil and store them. Obviously, if the soil is empty the plant will be empty.

The next phase of maturity for the plant is the production of vitamins, enzymes, and other nutrients. We usually call this the ripening period. The mature plant will produce these vital nutrients with sunlight and the process of photosynthesis. The ideal maturing process is referred to as vine ripening. It is this phase of development that gives the food the vitamins and minerals content. Each vitamin and mineral has one or more jobs, and they all work together for the good of the body that consumes them.

Now, think about this: plants grown in hungry soil and picked green, before ripening or making vitamins and other nutrients, have little or no nutritional value. This is why it can take more than 10,000 calories to get even the minimal amount of nutrition reflected in the RDA. Could it be that one of the reasons we are ill and obese is the fact that our food does not give us the essential nutrition our bodies need every day? Yes! And in addition to that deficiency of nutrition, we get an abundance of negatives from the chemicals and the after harvest processing.

Our food is chemically treated to prolong shelf life. It is irradiated because of the filthy conditions it is exposed to in the fields and warehouses. This irradiation, or electronic pasteurization, subjects the food to radiation equal to as much as a million chest x-rays. Many studies show that irradiation mutates the DNA of the food and changes its molecular structure. Anyone seeking to challenge this or to learn more will find it an easy web search.

Next, if the food is processed, there are hundreds of toxic chemicals that could be added to it. It is estimated that the average American consumes over nine pounds of toxic chemicals each year in the form of artificial colors, flavors, sweeteners and preservatives. This does not include the tons of herbicides and pesticides used to grow the food. To be sure crops can withstand the toxins that are sprayed on them, many of the crops we consume are genetically modified to withstand herbicides and actually contain the pesticides. Also, genetically engineered plants are shown to need more chemicals to protect them from pests. (As I said earlier there are deeper moral issues with genetic engineering. It involves crossing the genes of animals and vegetables to create life forms that never would have evolved in nature. This is worth considering for the savvy consumer, but is outside of the scope of this book.) Still I am compelled to include some findings that relate to overall health and perhaps impacts obesity.

Mike Adams, Health Ranger wrote in his post on September 21, 2012:

(NaturalNews) The GMO debate is over. There is no longer any legitimate, scientific defense of growing GM crops for human consumption. The only people still clinging to the outmoded myth that "GMOs are safe" are scientific mercenaries with financial ties to Monsanto and the biotech industry.

GMOs are an anti-human technology. They threaten the continuation of life on our planet. They are a far worse threat than terrorism, or even the threat of nuclear war.

*As a shocking new study has graphically shown, **GMOs are the new thalidomide**. When rats eat GMO corn they develop horrible tumors. Seventy percent of females die prematurely, and virtually all of them suffer severe organ damage from consuming GMO. These are the scientific conclusions of the first truly "long-term" study ever conducted on GMO consumption in animals, and the findings are absolutely horrifying. What this reveals is that **genetic engineering turns FOOD into POISON**.*

Remember thalidomide? Babies being born with no arms and other heart-breaking deformities? Thalidomide was pushed as "scientific" and "FDA approved." The same lies are now being told about GMO: they're safe. They're nutritious. They will feed the world!

*But the real science now coming out tells a different picture: **GMOs may be creating an entire generation of cancer victims** who have a frighteningly heightened risk of growing massive mammary gland tumors caused by the consumption of GM foods. We are witnessing what may turn out to be **the worst and most costly blunder in the history of western science**: the mass poisoning of billions of people with a toxic food crop that was never properly tested in the first place.*

A ten year study in Norway has shown conclusively that consuming genetically modified corn contributes to weight gain and obesity. The findings were published July 11, 2012 in Norway by Forskning.no, an online news source devoted to Norwegian and international research. Lead author] Professor Krogdahl explains: *"It has often been claimed that the new genes in genetically modified foods can't do any damage because all genes are broken down beyond recognition in the gut. Our results show the contrary; that genes can be taken up across the intestinal wall, is transferred to the blood and is left in the blood, muscle and liver in large chunks so that they can be easily recognized ... The biological impact of this gene transfer is unknown." "The results show a positive link between GE corn and obesity. Animals fed a GE corn diet got fatter quicker and retained the weight compared to animals fed a non-GE grain diet. The studies were performed on rats, mice, pigs and salmon, achieving the same results.*

... Researchers found distinct changes to the intestines of animals fed GMOs compared to those fed non-GMOs. This confirms other studies done by US researchers. Significant changes occurred in the digestive systems of the test animals' major organs including the liver, kidneys, pancreas, genitals and more."

For years those of us in natural health have followed our instincts and relied on non-conclusive studies and anecdotal profiles to sound an alarm against GMOs. Personally, it has been a question of morality. It is simply immoral to introduce genes across species lines that never would have occurred in nature. Pollination respects nature, genetic modification will destroy nature. More than any single person, Jeffery Smith has devoted his life to exposing the dangers of GMOs. For anyone wanting to know more he is an easy Google.

The only reason for genetic modification of seeds is the creation of intellectual property and the sale of toxins for use in food production. Many of the chemicals used in modern agriculture directly damage the brain and the central nervous system. Many others are called endocrine disrupters, because once inside the body they mimic the peptides and other hormones used by the organs to communicate. They interfere with metabolism, and they can and do contribute to obesity and ill health.

In September of 2012 Michael Taylor, MONSANTO'S VICE PRESIDENT, was appointed by President Obama to be a senior advisor to the commissioner of the FDA. This is the same man that was in charge of FDA policy when GMO's were allowed into the US food supply without undergoing a single test to determine their safety. He had been Monsanto's attorney before becoming policy chief at the FDA and then he became Monsanto's Vice President and chief lobbyist. Now he is back through the ***Revolving Door*** as the senior advisor to the commissioner of the FDA. Michael Taylor is **America's food safety czar.**

The Staff of Life, or A Stack of Lies?

We sing about our beautiful America. The purple mountain's majesty, the spacious skies, the fruited plains, and, of course, the amber waves of grain. Today those amber waves have become a dominant part of our not-so-beautiful American diet. While they are pleasing to the eye and a major part of our agricultural economy, excessive consumption of these grains is now a major reason for our national health problems that begin with overweight and obesity. Several million people are classified with "syndrome X," a group of health markers warning of heart disease, cancer, diabetes, arthritis and other inflammatory diseases.

Why? Simple.

We devote too much of our caloric intake to foods that produce storable fat, not energy. We have become an overweight, under-nourished nation with sky rocketing health care costs and a diminishing quality of life and health.

It does not have to be this way...

The Grain Controversy

While the government agencies dance around the issue of obesity and syndrome X, they do not recognize their own role in the development of the problem or take meaningful steps to promote change. The recent revisions in the USDA Food recommendations actually increased to 50% the amount of calories we should get from grains. The new recommendations did for the first time make a distinction between whole grains and refined grains. It suggests that half the grains consumed be whole grains. That might have been an improvement if it weren't for the increase in total grains.

You are probably asking, "What is wrong with grains?" Perhaps nothing. **In moderation.** We are the nation with the "amber waves of grain" right? I call them the "amber waves of gain." Weight gain. The grains the Bible refers to as the "Staff of Life" are not the same grains that we grow in much colder climates. In fact, the reason we are growing grains in a colder climate is because they will grow there, where other crops will not grow. When it comes to grain, America grows far more than it needs. In fact, the government gives tax money to the factory-farms to keep prices higher despite the surplus. Because grains will grow bountifully where other crops will not, and because grains offer a winter crop as well, we grow them. Since the USDA has created the surplus with our tax money, it now asks us to consume more grains that our bodies need. In other words, one hand washes the other and both hands get dirty.

Hybrid Vigor

A hundred years ago farming in the United States was far different from today's chemical laden, mechanized farming methods. We might also note that food related diseases were limited to scarcity and spoilage; there were no health challenges from eating the natural harvest. Hundreds of varieties of food crops were grown, including many strains of wheat. Wheat was still the Biblical staff of life. And other food crops came in many varieties and choices.

Some 250,000 edible plant species have been recorded. Of these, only about 200 have been cultivated for food crops. Most of the food on our planet comes from as few as 20 crops in only 8 food groups. Our basic food choices have been drastically reduced in the last one hundred years. That is a challenging statement when one considers the thousands of items found packed in the isles of our modern supermarkets.

The practice of saving seeds began to diminish in the 1940s with the discovery of hybrid vigor. It was discovered that seeds from plants that had been cross pollinated with cousin or grandparent plants would produce a more abundant harvest. Farmers began to rely on seed companies to make the pairings that produced a different family of seeds each year. Pollination is a natural and essential process and the strains grew stronger. The down side? Each year fewer and fewer varieties were offered, and the consumer had fewer and fewer choices at the market. Cabbage for example dropped from around a 500 varieties in 1900 to as few as 20 today. Wheat has experienced a similar narrowing, and the *Staff of Life* holds little resemblance to the wheat that was cultivated in Mesopotamia when farming began. The emphasis has been on developing stronger strains that will produce bigger harvests. We have learned to support these new seeds with chemicals and artificial fertilizers. Harvests are abundant. Nutrition is abysmal.

Perfect Poison

Dr. William Davis, a cardiologist says that wheat has evolved into a "perfect poison," and he says that wheat is at the center of our obesity epidemic. Davis said that the wheat we eat these days isn't the wheat your grandma had: "It's an 18-inch tall plant created by genetic research in the '60s and '70s. This thing has many new features nobody told you about, such as there's a new protein in this thing called gliadin. It's not gluten." Many people have trouble digesting gluten. It is the component that makes wheat products bind together. For example it is added to bagel flour to make them more chewy. Some people have gluten sensitivities that can present a host of health issues. Celiac disease is a more serious reaction to gluten. The inability to digest it allows it to form an obstruction in the small intestine blocking absorption of nutrients and producing conditions that can become extremely painful and life-threatening.

Dr. Davis says gliadin, the substance found in the new wheat, is an opiate. "This thing binds into the opiate receptors in your brain and in most people stimulates appetite, such that we consume 440 more calories per day, 365 days per year." Before we knew that processing the wheat isolated its fat making components, but if we ate *whole grains* the fiber delayed digestion and gave the body a chance to process it before adding to the fat stores. Davis says that eating whole grains is the same as smoking a filtered cigarette; it is just another degree of bad. Davis says dramatic weight loss is being recorded among people who drop all wheat from their diet. "We are seeing hundreds of thousands of people losing 30, 80, 150 pounds. Diabetics become no longer diabetic; people with arthritis having dramatic relief. People losing leg swelling, acid reflux. Irritable bowel syndrome, depression, and on and on every day." Dr. Davis has added gliadin to the list of reasons to avoid wheat, but gluten remains along with other documented problems with the grain that was once worthy of being called *The Staff of Life.*

Dangerous Grains

In their book, "Dangerous Grains", James Braly, M.D. and Ron Hoggan, M.A., list nearly 200 medical conditions that are associated with the consumption of large amounts of grains. These include obesity and other markers from **Syndrome X**, as well as several autoimmune conditions. They point out that many people have sensitivity to gluten. Gluten is a protein from the most common grains. It is not easily digested. Many people suffer great harm from this sensitivity that does not always show up in regular medical examinations. The answer for most people is a "Gluten Free Diet" that does not include wheat, oats, barley or rye. The undigested gluten gets into the body and its presence triggers an immune response that results in an inflammatory condition. (Oats grown in isolation from other gluten containing grains may be gluten free.)

Second Hand Grains

We use grains to fatten our meat and poultry animals for market. Grains do make fat, but grains also increase acidity. Fat and acidity lead to high blood pressure, oxygen deprivation, inflammatory conditions throughout the veins and bodies, and other markers for ill health and heart disease. If we can use grains to fatten cattle, what happens to us when we eat the same grains? Or, what happens to us when we consume the meat and poultry fattened on grains. Cattle thrive on grass, not the seeds. When we eat meat and dairy products from animals that are pasture fed, there is a world of difference. Beef and other pasture fed animals have less than 10% saturated fat, have a pH near the desired 7.2 and are rich in essential fatty acids.

When these same animals are placed in feeding pens, filled with antibiotics and growth hormones, they produce a completely different product, a fat one. The saturated fat is now as high as 70% with little or no essential fatty acids. The acid level is off the chart. Grass is alkaline forming when digested and grains are acid forming. As we eat these growth hormones we must ask, "If they made the animal fat, what will they do to us?" Aside from the toxic laden fat, the growth hormone is rBGH, a genetically modified substance from anthrax pathogens, that is linked to several forms of cancer in European research. The countries of the EU and several other countries refuse U.S. beef imports because of the use of rBGH. Some of those are Third World countries with serious food shortages. It is banned in every industrialized nation on earth, except the U.S., Canada, Mexico and Brazil.

rBGH is made from genetically modified anthrax germs. Developed by Monsanto in the late 80s it was found to both increase weight gain and milk production when given to cattle. An ear clip on a beef cow will add substantial dollars to the value of the animal. If the clip is illegally attached to the rump of the animal, it will add even more dollars to its value. There are no restrictions on the amount of rBGH that can be used on a dairy cow. When Monsanto was bringing it to market the FDA asked for a scientific report. The company had a report in its files that had been prepared by one of the scientists working on the project, Margaret Miller. Miller had left Monsanto to take a position with the FDA; the **Revolving Door** swings again. She was Deputy Director of Human Food Safety and Consultative Services, New Animal Drug Evaluation Office, Center for Veterinary Medicine in the United States Food and Drug Administration. Guess who reviewed the "science" report from Monsanto? The same Margaret Miller who wrote it a couple of years earlier when she was on the Monsanto payroll (directly). It was approved with the trade name of Posilac.

There is another second hand issue with eating meat and poultry, antibiotics. It was discovered that animals given sub therapeutic doses antibiotics would reach their mature weight in almost half the time. Although some modifications have been made in recent times, for years the greater percentage of antibiotics produced in the United States were used by the ton for spiking the grains used to fatten meat animals for market. Funny thing about Mother Nature, if she does not make it, she will not take it back. All those tons of antibiotics remained in the meat, or were excreted to eventually become a permanent part of Earth's water resources. Either way we ingested those tons of antibiotics. What happened? Superbugs. Drug resistant germs that stalk us in our hospitals and other healthcare facilities. MRSA, a drug resistant form of staff, is killing more people than Aids according to the Centers for Disease Control. The agency also reports that once conquered diseases such as tuberculosis are back and stronger. Our concern here is obesity, and again: if it makes the animals fat, it can make us fat.

Our Pets and Our Pocketbooks

In addition to providing us with an abundance of non-nutrition, grains are also used to make dog and cat food. Where or when in nature did the carnivores start grazing? Does feeding grains to meat eating animals have an impact on their health? Do we really need a scientific study, to answer that question? This is another illustration of the point I am making with this book. We consume what is abundant, not what is nutritious and needed by our bodies. Animal feed is simply another opportunity to use the surplus of grains created by our tax dollars. The makers of animal feed save money and make higher profits. Meanwhile, we have to spend more to pay our pet's veterinary bills for the same reason we pay more to our doctors and others in healthcare. Cheap food is not cheap when you add up the associated costs. The costs are important, but quality of life is more important. We do not commit to our pets to save money at the expense of their quality of life. We want more for them than unnatural grains and by-products which can be anything from feces to scraps from the floor of the slaughter house.

But Eating American is Cheap!

One of the few excuses offered for the standard American Diet is that it is cheap. If you call a .99 cent cheeseburger cheap, you should realize how much the fries and soda are costing you, especially when you take advantage of the super-size "deal." You might be paying over a dollar for half a potato presented as French fries, and the big soda costs less to produce than the cup it is in. In fact, the biggest cost in selling soda is the containers. A case of 1,000 16 oz. cups will cost well under $100.00 or less than ten cents. Carbonated water, ice and a squirt of syrup will cost about the same. That is why they can break even on the burger and make big profits on sodas and fries. We are lulled into the fantasy of cheap food in our country. But to understand cost and value, we have to look beyond the price paid at the checkout counter. If we knew how much of our tax money was spent getting a food item to the grocery shelf, we might not think it so cheap.

So many costs that have to do with the standard American diet have yet to be compounded:

- How much does it cost us through government to clean up the chemicals used in producing our food?
- How much tax money is spent to subsidize and create a surplus of cheap food?
- How much more tax money goes to the well-connected political figures who provide storage for our food surpluses?
- What is the long term cost of consuming chemically-laden food measured in terms of healthcare costs and lost wages?
- What are the long range healthcare costs of nutritional deficiencies and obesity?

Aside from the fact that cheap food is not really cheap, there is a far deeper public issue. What does this kind of food cost us in terms of energy, vitality and quality of life? There is no measure for these intangible treasures of life. The next time you think or hear someone say, "Organic food costs too much," advise them to look at the big picture. Or look at how much organic food can save you in healthcare costs and quality of life issues. Junk food is kept cheap by tax supported subsidies through the Farm Bill and other giveaways. On the surface food stamps appear to be a humanitarian effort, other of us see it as another subsidy for the food manufacturers that make the products approved for purchase. Try using food stamps at the weekly farmers market, or to buy a share in a community garden.

Time Magazine, June 23, 2008 reported in a series of articles on childhood obesity that the cost of fresh fruits and vegetables rose between 1989 and 2005 by 74.6%. During that same period *Time* reported there was a reduction in the cost of junk and fatty foods of 26.5%. If we want to do something about the run-away healthcare costs that are draining our pockets and our national treasury we could begin with the costly subsidies that promote health-wrecking food. Would that be a win-win?

I offer one case in point on what poor quality foods are costing us. A study published in the *Journal of Psychiatry* found that children who were deficient in only four essential nutrients were more likely to become criminals. Those missing zinc, B vitamins, iron and protein were found to be more aggressive and antisocial by the age of 8, by 41%. At 17 years of age they were 51% more likely to be antisocial and engage in criminal behavior. It costs us often as much as $100,000 per year to house an inmate in our prison system. What would be the long-range savings if only half of these inmates had dietary supplements and a better diet as children? If we could cut our prison costs by 50%, we could probably educate every child in America kindergarten through graduate school, **without a school tax.**

Granted, criminal activity is an extreme example. Let me give you a less challenging image. Think about the obese, depressed and defocused woman next to you in the supermarket checkout line. Look at the soda, chips, snacks, treats, and "cheap food" in her cart.

Does she have to suffer through her life ashamed of her appearance and never knowing God's full intention for her? Look at the underweight, defocused, sad-faced child with deep, dark circles under the eyes salivating for the snacks. What does this little person have to look forward to? I hope not prison or the legacy of his or her parents.

Any way we look at it, cheap food is not cheap! If it costs you your health, it certainly is not cheap. Remember this, "You cannot buy back your health at any price".

Is High Protein the Answer?

Often, people on one of the popular high protein diets consume large amounts of fatty meats. I have often wondered if they realized that the fat produced by grains can metabolize the same as carbohydrates. Commercial meat, dairy, poultry and even farm raised fish are, as it were, a form of grains because of what they are fed within the factory farming system. They come to us with much higher amounts of fat to convert to glucose and subsequently to body fat. They increase our acidity. And they add antibiotics to our toxic body burden. Again, if grains and chemicals make the animal fat, what happens to us when we eat the animal? Yes! Fat on top of fat equals more fat!

In fact, a keen eye can glean the effects of the food-that-makes-us-eat-more-food phenomenon at every level. For instance, the government has proposed that every child have a full hour of vigorous activity each day to burn off some of the extra pounds. At the risk of sounding cynical, my first image was not youngsters at play. My first image was a computerized report estimating the extra dollars the activity would produce in added caloric intake. In fact, exercise is the only thing that seems to have a consensus in Washington. The only way to increase food consumption is to promote more physical activity.

Every time there is a suggestion that people eat less or make better food choices, the grocery, restaurant and related lobbies object. Obviously they are trying to protect their income. That is their job. It is the job of the regulators to protect us, but it is pretty clear who pulls their strings. Like most Americans, I am tired of being told that exercise is the answer to our health problems. It is true that we spend less time chasing balls and more time surfing the Web or the "boob-tube." Still, gyms have never had more members. Sports equipment sales have never been better. You see people running everywhere. Golf courses are packed, so are the swimming pools and tennis courts. Most people walk two or three miles shopping at a big mall.

I think exercise is excellent for the human body. I also think many people are using exercise to their own detriment. I know some people who are at the gym almost every day, but they are eating more junk and drinking more alcohol thinking they can burn it off. Actually, many people are accelerating their aging process with excessive exercise. Every time we burn energy at the cell level, we release free radicals and Homocystein. Free radicals are associated with oxidative damage to healthy cells. Homocystein, causes thickening of the arteries and is associated with such things as heart disease, colon cancer and Alzheimer's. The amino acid, cystein stimulates growth along with other amino acids. Homo, or lone, cystein causes growth in the wrong place and without natural moderators. If people who engage in vigorous exercise do not increase their antioxidants and B Vitamins, they can suffer oxidative damage and develop inflammation in their veins. When those who are overweight and poorly nourished begin more vigorous activity, they can severely stress themselves into a more severe condition. That said, I am reminded that cautious exercise can begin to improve metabolism and several health markers among the overweight population. I also am led to challenge the concept of "no pain, no gain". Pain is the body's way of telling us when we are overstressing. Pain means stop.

We need a balance of nutrition, rest, meditation, fresh air, pure water and exercise. We suffer without **all** of these things—and exercise alone is not the answer.

☙❧

Health and Proper pH Balance

I want to tell you more about pH, the potential for Hydrogen. It is a means of measuring the alkaline or acid levels of the body. It is a scale of 0 to 14, and the desired reading for a healthy human is 7.2.

I recall our first swimming pool. As a young couple we were excited to have a place for the children and ourselves to swim and cool off right in the back yard. The excitement faded on the third day when we woke to a green pool. We added more chlorine (that was before we learned that there were other ways to keep a pool clear). Shortly we were out of chlorine and the pool was a deeper green. I took a sample of water to the pool store. The clerk put the sample in the machine for analysis. The machine reported the need for one of everything produced by the company that supplied machine. I went home with a trunk load of chemicals and instructions on how to use them. I treated the green water carefully following the instructions. Next morning the water was a darker shade of green. For several days, I scoured the countryside for the magic chemical to make the water clear. Every day it was a deeper shade of green. Finally, I heard about pH. I checked the pH and it was too acid. I added 3 big boxes of baking soda. It was incredible. Within in an hour the water was crystal clear.

The human body is much like a swimming pool, in that it is a closed environment. When the pH is off, I can visualize the green stuff building and choking off oxygen. In the early 1930s cancer was induced in more than two dozen test animals by causing their acid levels to rise. When the oxygen is choked out by the acid, it is an active environment for carbon-loving cancer cells. High acid contributes to everything from hair loss and gastric distress to autoimmune diseases as well as cancer. At the same time if the body becomes too alkaline it can host bacteria and fungus. Balance again is the key to health. Garden fresh food supports a balanced pH in the body. Processed food increases the probability of a high acid condition.

⌒⌒

The American Diet

The United States Department of Agriculture reports that Americans get most of their daily calories from: **Milk, colas, white bread, sugar, ground beef, white flour products, and processed American cheese food.** As we know, these foods are loaded with trans fatty acids, sugar or high fructose corn syrup and chemicals. The Government topped its own famous Food Pyramid with the smallest triangle representing fats and sweets, warning us to "use sparingly." The same basic recommendations have been continued in the pie and other graphics used by the USDA. But what about all the fats and sugars found in the categories before one reaches the pyramid's top? Through all of the most recent decades under Republican and Democratic administrations the story has not changed. Each year sees more *Revolving Door* decisions concerning the food we are promoted to consume, and each year we have grown more obese. Until there is a policy change we will continue to suffer more health failures and go deeper in debt to finance a system that eventually will kill us.

We are obsessed with food. Food occupies entire television channels; diets consume billions of dollars yearly; and cookbooks sell like hotcakes. We are growing fatter, but health statistics prove that we are malnourished. The numbers of deaths from diseases that reflect dietary deficiencies continue to rise. Obviously we need a new focus on nutrition because what we are doing does not work. As early as 1978 the US Surgeon General estimated that more than 75% of disease related deaths in the United States were connected to diet.

And yet we love food—the way it tastes and the way it feels when we chew and swallow it. We experience many sensations of the tongue, but very little real flavor. It is the roof of the mouth or the pallet that senses flavors. The tongue reacts only to sweet, sour, salt and bitter. It also reacts to creamy. Crunchy is another mouth sensation that is flavorless, but has become a desirable trait for some foods. We should also add heat to this list of sensations. Many people love the sensation of hot peppers and seek a hot pepper experience from their food. Foods that cater to these sensations often are the ones that contain the least nutrition. Many people are so accustomed to the sensations of the tongue that they have no experience with real flavors, like those from the foods themselves, or the enhancements of herbs and spices.

We mentioned earlier that most Americans get the bulk of their calories from milk, sugar, colas, white bread, ground beef, white flour and processed cheese food. Add to that a few tons of mined salt reconstituted with mined iodine and a few thousand gallons of refined, degenerative oils, and we discover that we are trying to live on negative nutrients.

Let us take a look at the foods that are supplying most of our calories:

Milk: Does It Do a Body Good?

Milk contains saturated animal fat, some calcium and an insignificant amount of synthetic Vitamin D. Actually, if it were not homogenized, it would be the more nutritious food in this group. If it were raw, not pasteurized, it would be a nutritious food. The European dietary intake of dairy is far greater than that of the United States, yet their incidence of heart disease and other illnesses generally related to high fat consumption is much lower.

The pasteurization process is different in Europe and the milk is not homogenized. Cheese, yogurt and other dairy products are aged the natural way. The American way is to speed it through a factory process with chemical additives to yield higher profits and longer shelf life. In other words, it is a different kind of dairy product. Actually the Europeans reject American milk products because of the growth hormones we use to increase the cows' milk production.

Another factor that we must address is the use of antibiotics among cattle in dairy herds. Cattle used for dairy production and for meats live in filthy conditions. Dairy cows in some milking operations are never turned out to green pasture. They spend their days in crowded barns waiting their twice per day turn at the milking station. The bigger operations milk 24/7. Beef cattle are held in crowded pens while they are fattened standing in feces and urine. Hogs are housed in multi-story facilities with the feces and urine draining from the top levels down thru every story to the bottom. The stress tends to increase the animals appetite for additional weight gain.

Additionally, the soy and corn oils in their diet reduces their immune levels. In an effort to keep the cattle from infecting each other with diseases, they are continuously given sub-therapeutic doses of antibiotics. Trace amounts of these antibiotics are found in dairy products according to the USDA's own Inspector General. No studies have been published on the long-term effects of ingesting these products, but it is believed that they compromise healthy gut flora and provide an environment that encourages bacteria to mutate in the body and become resistant to antibiotics.

Another drawback of milk is that it contains lactose, a 12-carbon sugar. Glucose has only six carbons in its molecule. The body has to split the lactose molecule into one of glucose and one of galactose. Galactose is an inflammatory agent and causes phlegm to collect in the sinus cavities and elsewhere. Lactose as a sugar adds to the sugar burden of the body. Many weight-conscious people use skim milk or reduced fat milk to avoid the calories. Skim milk contains the same amount of lactose as whole milk, and they are equally fattening in that regard.

Once the milk is pasteurized, most of its better nutrients including calcium are locked out of the digestive process. That's right, we do not get the calcium we think we are getting from pasteurized dairy products. For that matter cutting edge science tells us that the body does not maintain bone mass from dietary calcium. The body makes the calcium it uses for bone mass from magnesium, the center element of chlorophyll. That is why leafy greens are good for your bones. (Read my book, *Bless My Bones* if you want to follow up this point.)

The government nationalized the milk business years ago. Dairy farming is one of the few businesses one can go into with a guaranteed customer for the product. That does not mean that all dairy farmers prosper. The price of milk is determined by a small town in Wisconsin. A dairy farmer in other parts of the country may not see the same profits as the farmers in Wisconsin or other less expensive states. What does the government do with all that milk? It makes it into powdered skim milk and rents a storage facility from a politically connected "fat cat" where it stays for several months. Then it is sold back to the milk bottling industry. Skim milk you buy is probably reconstituted powder coming out of storage at a bargain price. Did you get it for a bargain? Did you think it came from a cow hours before your purchase?

The surplus milk that does not go into powdered storage is made into processed cheese food and stored by another "fat cat" until there is no more storage space; then, it goes to the food programs or is sold at a bargain price for the consumer market. More on processed cheese food later. For those who like milk and cheese. Look for raw or unpasteurized products. That would be naturally aged cheese products. It is not that easy to find unprocessed milk. Organic milk products tend to be hormone and antibiotic free, although they are pasteurized. Now it is time to talk about sugar and other sweeteners.

A Spoonful of Sugar?

This entire book and ten more could be written on sweeteners and their negative impact on our weight and health. I will try to be brief, but we have to address this tongue sensation that is killing us.

We must make a distinction here between raw sugar and refined sugar. Usually when we refer to sugar we are talking about the refined white stuff that dominates our diets. Sugar in moderation is not the problem, unless a person has diabetes or hypoglycemia. However, sugar becomes a problem when it is consumed in quantities that exceed the body's needs and ability to metabolize it.

It is the refining of sugar that causes many of our health problems. When raw sugar is refined into those pretty white crystals, it is stripped of its natural proteins and fibers. It is refined because it is easier to store, easier to package, and it dissolves more quickly. In other words, sugar is more profitable in its refined form for those who sell and use large amounts of it processing foods or beverages.

However, in its refined form sugar no longer contains the natural elements needed for simple digestion. These nutrients need digestion, and the digestive process gives the body time to prepare for its entry and conversion to energy. Refined white sugar with no nutrition requires no digestion and enters the body almost immediately. The glycemic process stresses the pancreas and the liver. Eventually, according to the available literature, repeated and excessive ingestion of sugar can lead to insulin resistance and diabetes.

The most common kind of sugar is sucrose (table sugar) which is an unnatural, refined sweetener and a 12-carbon molecule. Eating a whole food that contains a 12-carbon sugar is natural; refining and concentrating makes it unnatural. Remember, glucose is a 6-carbon molecule. Sucrose in the body must be converted to one molecule of glucose and another of fructose, sometimes called grape sugar. The refined sugar may enter the body more quickly than the system can prepare for its utilization. The glucose may be turned to fat before it can be used for energy, while the second 6-carbon molecule will most likely go directly to fat. Sucrose has the potential to make twice the glucose, or twice the fat, that would be made from fructose or honey.

Table sugar can cause spikes in serum blood sugar. This excess of blood sugar, in addition to stressing the liver and pancreas, can also disrupt the endocrine glands, since the adrenals secret adrenaline to control the sugar overload. This secretion of adrenaline can contribute to anxiety in adults and hyperactivity in children. Levels of sugar in the blood are now used as a marker for potential heart disease along with cholesterol and other tradition markers. Recent studies also show that there is a direct relationship between the amount of insulin produced in a person's body and longevity. The more insulin produced in the body, the shorter the lifespan.

In a healthy person, the liver and pancreas use glucose to form glycogen energy stores. During the periods between meals these stores are used to maintain a constant energy level. Fat is not always an energy store. Actually, as these refined carbohydrates are converted to fat, they take more energy and nutrients from the body than they deliver. These are worse than empty calories; they are negative nutrients. It takes even more energy to carry them around as fat.

Most Americans at one time consumed between 100 and 150 pounds of refined sugar per year. The amount of sugar consumed today is about half the amount from a few years ago. The reduction in sugar does not signal an improvement, however. The amount of high fructose corn syrup, HFCS, consumed today is equal to, or slightly higher than the amount of sugar once consumed per person. In other words, the sugar has been replaced by a potentially more harmful sweetener. Actually a greater percentage of sweet commercial products today are made with HFCS. Consuming large amounts of either sugar or HFCS can cause the body to become clogged with glucose. The liver and pancreas reach their limit of glycogen production. Once the capacity is reached the excess is turned into fat and stored.

Imagine a vehicle with a gasoline engine and an expandable gas tank. If the tank is filled with more fuel than the engine is burning, eventually the expanding tank will be as big as the vehicle itself. If we continue to consume more calories than we can burn, eventually our fat stores will dominate our body.

We use our fresh glycogen for energy during the day, and we store the excess as a little more fat. As this glucose is made into fat for storage it begins to clog more than the space between our cells. It begins to compromise our immune system and our health long range. It is estimated that the sweetener in a can of soda will reduce one's immune level by one-third. That would mean that a person who drinks three sodas per day has virtually no immunity.

Refined sugar and other refined carbohydrates drain the body of necessary minerals and reduce the intestinal ability to digest and produce vitamins. These sweeteners also cause the release of "free calcium"; this is the form of calcium that makes stones and clogs joints and arteries.

Sugar and other so-called quick carbohydrates increase free radical activity in the body which can also lower immune response and accelerate aging. Dr. Paresh Dandona from the State University of New York at Buffalo writing in the August, 2000 *Journal of Clinical Endocrinology and Metabolism* reported that excess sugar in the blood increases production of free radicals and depletes the body of important antioxidant vitamins, such as vitamin E.

Fourteen healthy people were given 75 MG of pure glucose (that would be the same amount contained in two cans of most sodas); the second group of six healthy people were given a solution with no glucose. Blood samples one hour later in the glucose group showed a significant increase in free radical activity. Two hours later the free radical activity doubled. This explains the earlier report that claimed that three cans of soda can wipe out the immune system. It appears that the sugar load simply uses up the body's antioxidant vitamins and other important antioxidants such as glutathione, considered the cornerstone of the immune system. The Buffalo study clearly indicates why the obese are prone to various illnesses and why diabetics are prone to heart disease and circulatory disorders.

HFCS is a liquid and is easier to store and use than sugar. It is sweeter than sugar and easier to blend into products. Above all, it is cheaper than sugar. Despite what you may have heard, your body does know the difference between old fashioned sugar and HFCS. HFCS has a different digestive pattern than sugar and in many ways can be more harmful to the body. It enters the body as half glucose and half unbound fructose. The glucose needs no digestion and confronts the pancreas too quickly with a challenge to the blood sugar levels. At the same time, the unbound fructose causes hormonal disruptions. Fructose, fruit sugar, digests differently when it is isolated from the fibers of a fruit.

Unbound fructose tampers with our hormones by first suppressing the insulin needed for its own processing plus that needed for the glucose. Over time this leads to insulin resistance at the cellular level. The HFCS disrupts the hormone that controls fat making, leptin, forcing the body to convert the glucose to fat. The next activity of the HFCS causes a secretion of a stomach hormone, ghrelin, which triggers hunger. Yes, drinking or eating something with HFCS will make you hungry when your body does not need food. For more, see Dr Nancy Appleton's book, *Lick the Sugar Habit,* which presents a thorough review of the harms traceable to this and other sugar forms.

In 1900 only one person in thirty died from cancer. Heart disease was not the number one killer; most people died of old age. Only those who were uprooted by political abuses died young. The 12-carbon sugars were not part of the human diet on a large scale until the turn of the century. Before that time the refining process was done by hand and it was very expensive. Only rich people could eat refined carbohydrates. Therefore, cancer, heart disease and diabetes were diseases reserved for the wealthy.

The industrial revolution brought these refined foods to the masses. Today everybody is expected to have some kind of heart disease, and one in three, not thirty, will have of cancer. (There is one report that has the cancer incidence very close to one in every two people.) So the Industrial Revolution brought sickness to the masses with its refined foods.

Today, the wealthy eat more expensive organic foods and hire personal nutritionists to keep them from eating refined foods, while the poor and middle classes eat the poisonous refined foods that are so readily available and more affordable. At one time, this information about the ills of refined sugars and carbohydrates was nonexistent, but now it is abundant. Information on the ills of smoking is also abundant. But bad habits are hard to break.

Obesity in American has been on the rise since the introduction of refined sugar to the market, but the figures exploded when HFCS came into use. Just to review:

It hampers insulin production by slapping the body with a load of fructose and glucose.

It stimulates fat making because of the impact on leptin.

It stimulates hunger by impacting ghrelin.

HFCS makes you hungry and in even modest amounts will add weight to your body. One other note: leptin is a catalyst to other hormones including estrogen and reproductive hormones. It is suspect in some studies of pernicious puberty.

More recent research has added more than fat to the fire. The way the body is forced to process unbound fructose is as challenging as excessive alcohol consumption. When we eat fruit, the fructose is bound to the fibers of the fruit and the digestive process is not challenged. When we consume fructose as a juice or as HFCS there is a different set of circumstances for the body to handle.

According to Dr. Robert Lustig, Professor of Pediatrics in the Division of Endocrinology at the University of California, fructose is a "chronic, dose-dependent liver toxin." And just like alcohol, fructose is metabolized directly into *fat*–not cellular energy. His paper on the topic was published in the *Journal of the Academy of Nutrition and Dietetics*,[1] Dr. Lustig explains the three similarities between fructose and its fermentation byproduct, ethanol (alcohol):

1. Your liver's metabolism of fructose is similar to alcohol, as they both serve as substrates for converting dietary carbohydrate into fat, which promotes insulin resistance, dyslipidemia (abnormal fat levels in the bloodstream), and fatty liver

2. Fructose undergoes the Maillard reaction with proteins, leading to the formation of superoxide free radicals that can result in liver inflammation similar to acetaldehyde, an intermediary metabolite of ethanol

3. By "stimulating the 'hedonic pathway' of the brain both directly and indirectly," Dr. Lustig noted, "fructose creates habituation, and possibly dependence; also paralleling ethanol."

Dr. Lustig concluded:

"Thus, fructose induces alterations in both hepatic [liver] metabolism and central nervous system energy signaling, leading to a 'vicious cycle' of excessive consumption and disease consistent with metabolic syndrome. On a societal level, the treatment of fructose as a commodity exhibits market similarities to ethanol. Analogous to ethanol, societal efforts to reduce fructose consumption will likely be necessary to combat the obesity epidemic."

Now, does your body know the difference? If anything clearly demonstrates government's role in our obesity, HFCS and its defense is clear. Here is a passage from the website put up to refute Dr Lustig:

There is <u>no scientific evidence that high fructose corn syrup is to blame for obesity and diabetes</u>. In fact, the U.S. Department of Agriculture data shows that consumption of high fructose corn syrup has actually been declining while obesity and diabetes rates continued to rise. Around the world, obesity levels are also rising even though HFCS consumption is limited outside of the U.S. Many other factors contribute to rising obesity levels including changes in lifestyle, diet and exercise and are unrelated to HFCS.

A complete expose of the history of HFCS is outside the mission of this book, but it is filled with well-known political figures who are deeply involved in the production and marketing of corn.

⌒⌒

How About Those Artificial Sweeteners?

Let us take a look at the most used artificial sweetener, a product that failed as a rat poison, but wound up being sold as a sugar replacement–aspartame. There is mounting evidence concerning the negative impact artificial sweeteners have on those who consume them regularly. For example, aspartame promotes sugar cravings that actually drive a person to consume the very calories he or she is trying to avoid. There is a risk of seizure associated with aspartame. It breaks into methanol in the digestive process. Methanol is the stuff in moonshine that can lead to blindness. Aspartame is an excitotoxin, because it can over excite brain cells and neurotransmission receptors, causing them to literally explode. The FDA has known for several years that aspartame can cause brain damage, tumors, seizures and neurological disorders. One might wonder why aspartame is still on the market. One might assume that the FDA having financed the development of it could influence its protection of aspartame.

On two occasions if have been approached by parents whose daughters were passing out or having seizures while away at college. They were not related, except by the cause of their daughters' problems. In both cases the girls were consuming large amounts of diet soda. They were suffering the effects of the aspartame.

There was a teller at the bank I have used for years. She was one who obviously struggled with her weight. She was found dead at home, and there was no obvious cause. I believe she consumed a toxic amount of aspartame. I asked about her and was told that she constantly sipped diet soda. Dr. Russell Blaylock has studied and written extensively about aspartame as a neurotoxin and documents several cases of death from excessive consumption of aspartame.

Yes. Aspartame came to us through the **Revolving Door.** According to the Norfolk Genetic Information Network:

"In 1985 Monsanto purchased G.D. Searle, the chemical company that held the patent to aspartame, the active ingredient in NutraSweet. Monsanto was apparently untroubled by aspartame's clouded past, including a 1980 FDA Board of Inquiry, comprised of three independent scientists, which confirmed that it "might induce brain tumors."

The FDA had actually banned aspartame based on this finding, only to have Searle Chairman Donald Rumsfeld (the former Secretary of Defense) vow to "call in his markers," to get it approved.

On January 21, 1981, the day after Ronald Reagan's inauguration, Searle re-applied to the FDA for approval to use aspartame in food as a sweetener, and Reagan's new FDA commissioner, Arthur Hayes Hull, Jr., appointed a 5-person Scientific Commission to review the board of inquiry's decision.

It soon became clear that the panel would uphold the ban by a 3-2 decision, but Hull then installed a sixth member on the commission, and the vote became deadlocked. He then personally broke the tie in aspartame's favor."

The newer artificial sweetener, Splenda, is actually made from sugar. To quote one of its chief detractors, Dr. Joseph Mercola, "It is made from sugar the same way gasoline is made from plants." They add chlorine to the sugar, which allows for a sweet taste on the way down, but inside the digestive system the chlorine keeps it from digesting. This combination creates a chlorocarbon. Personally, I am not comfortable with chlorine in my digestive system. I think it must harm the good gut flora, the good bacteria needed for good digestion and active immunity. The chlorine is bound to the sugar molecules with a synthetic bond similar to the ones used in the production of DDT and Agent Orange. The body has no mechanism for breaking these bonds.

Only limited information about the long-term use of Splenda has been made available. These small studies showed atrophy of the thymus gland (40%) and a compromised immune system. I also remember that all of the other artificial sweeteners were "safe" when they first came to market. Sorry, but I have grown distrustful of the system of regulation and approval.

The Cola Degeneration

There is little or nothing to redeem the consumption of colas, in my opinion. The sugar or HFCS content is about one third. And if the cola is sugar free, it is probably worse for you. In addition to the sweeteners, soda contains carbon bubbles. Why would a person whose body depends on plenty of oxygen to feed the cells fill himself or herself with carbon? Carbon is the stuff the body gives off as waste material. Yet, it is estimated that there are three million soda machines in the United States, many of them in schools.

Sodas do not help your bones either. The body is genetically programmed to keep a balance between phosphorus and calcium. Studies show that when we drink sodas and other carbonated beverages rich in phosphoric acid, the body is forced to surrender bone mass to achieve the pH balance. This depletes the calcium stores and bone mass. The link between osteoporosis and phosphorous intake is well established. So far, there is only a casual connection established between phosphorus intake and loss of calcium stores as it relates to muscle cramping and arrhythmia, or erratic heartbeat. When I hear about a person who has developed kidney stones, the first question I have is "how much soda have they been drinking?" When the calcium comes off the bone, it does not go back to the bone. It collects in the kidneys, joints or other part of the body.

Remember the swimming pool? Soda is a 2.5 on the acid/alkaline scale. It is estimated that it would take a dozen 8 oz glasses of water to neutralize the acid from one 12 oz soda.

Caffeine in soda has also become an issue. Researchers at Johns Hopkins University School of Medicine accused the bottling industry of adding caffeine to sodas to make them addictive. The industry criticized the study as poor science and claimed that the caffeine was used to enhance flavor. Roland Griffin, who led the study, however, said that the subjects could not taste the caffeine until they were given twice the amount allowed by the FDA. The Johns Hopkins group concluded, "We know adults and children can become physiologically and psychologically dependent on caffeinated soft drinks and experience a withdrawal syndrome if they stop consuming them."

In 1998, American consumption of soda was 585 cans per person. This explains why a seven-passenger family vehicle often has fourteen cup holders. Consumption of soda and other sweetened beverages is far greater today—and I would say, out of control.

At least there is recognition of the fact that consumption of large amounts of soda and other sweetened drinks contributes to weight gain. New York City has decided to limit the sale of these beverages to 16 oz. It is generally believed that those addicted will simply buy two and consume 32 ounces instead of 20. The problem is deeply seated in Washington and it is pervasive in food and beverages. That is where we will eventually be forced to make the changes. Unfortunately, our national debt may exceed our gross national product before we begin to chip away at the political infrastructure and culture of corruption that has the strangle hold on our connection to the Earth—our food.

There Is Another Excitotoxin Messing With Our Waistlines

MSG, monosodium glutamate, was developed in Japan shortly after WWII. It was first marketed in the United States as a meat tenderizer under the name of Accent. We all had a shaker near the stove. It was soon learned that a sprinkle of Accent on left overs or salad would freshen the flavor. Actually, MSG plays tricks on our taste buds by making everything taste good or better. Today MSG is used by the ton in the making of processed food and snacks. It can become addictive. It does make things taste better, or at least it makes us perceive them as tasting better.

There are a couple of problems with MSG. First, it is an obesity trigger. When scientists need fat rats for experiments, they simple feed them some MSG and they become obese. Second, it is a neurotoxin. Aspartame as we saw earlier is a neurotoxin. Aspartic acid carries impulses from the brain to our muscles. In excessive amounts the brain cells and receptors are over-excited and they literally burst. MSG is the opposite. Glutamic acid slows down brain function. Studies show that the amount of MSG one gets from a meal of Chinese food will dull the brain and lowered the IQ. We have enough to challenge brain function in this world without a neurotoxin mascaraing as a food enhancer dumbing us down even more.

MSG is an early example of the ***Revolving Door.*** Corruption of governmental and scientific committees by the food industry was disclosed in the late 1960s and early 1970s. In an article in the journal *Science* (1972), it was revealed that the National Academy of Sciences

(NAS) Food Protection Committee was being funded by the food, chemical and packaging industries. The U.S. Food and Drug Administration was relying on the NAS Committee for 'independent' information. The Chairman of the NAS Subcommittee investigating monosodium glutamate (MSG) had recently taken part in research partially funded by the MSG manufacturer. Another member of the Subcommittee became a spokesperson for the MSG industry. (*Science* 1972) Other members of the Subcommittee had ties to the MSG industry. Since that time numerous governmental committees have been corrupted by the placement of food industry-funded consultants on these committees."

Do not be fooled when the label says "no MSG." There are many other names for monosodium glutamate that are allowed to be listed as an ingredient without being identified as MSG. According to the Truth in Labeling website:

Names of ingredients that always contain processed free glutamic acid:

Glutamic acid (E 620)[2], Glutamate (E 620)
Monosodium glutamate (E 621)
Monopotassium glutamate (E 622)
Calcium glutamate (E 623)
Monoammonium glutamate (E 624)
Magnesium glutamate (E 625)
Natrium glutamate
Yeast extract
Anything "hydrolyzed"
Any "hydrolyzed protein"
Calcium caseinate, Sodium caseinate
Yeast food, Yeast nutrient
Autolyzed yeast
Gelatin
Textured protein
Soy protein, soy protein concentrate
Soy protein isolate
Whey protein, whey protein concentrate
Whey protein isolate
Anything "protein"
Vetsin
Ajinomoto

Names of ingredients that often contain or produce processed free glutamic acid:

Carrageenan (E 407)
Bouillon and broth
Stock
Any "flavors" or "flavoring"
Maltodextrin
Citric acid, Citrate (E 330)
Anything "ultra-pasteurized"
Barley malt
Pectin (E 440)
Protease
Anything "enzyme modified"
Anything containing "enzymes"
Malt extract
Soy sauce
Soy sauce extract
Anything "protein fortified"
Anything "fermented"
Seasonings

(1)   Glutamic acid found **in unadulterated protein** does not cause adverse reactions. To cause adverse reactions, the glutamic acid must have been processed/manufactured or come from protein that has been fermented.

The following are ingredients suspected of containing or creating sufficient processed free glutamic acid to serve as MSG-reaction triggers in HIGHLY SENSITIVE people:

Corn starch
Corn syrup
Modified food starch
Lipolyzed butter fat
Dextrose
Rice syrup
Brown rice syrup
Milk powder
Reduced fat milk (skim; 1%; 2%)
Most things low fat or no fat
Anything enriched
Anything vitamin enriched

The regulations allowing the use of MSG without clearly identifying it on the ingredient label were crafted by the manufacturers and rubber stamped by the **Revolving Door** regulators. Just one more way **"...the Government makes us fat."**

White Bread—Refined to the Max

If you are like me, you find it an insult to your intelligence to see the USDA's Food Pyramid or similar graphic on a package of white bread. That bread is as far removed from being a whole grain as I am from my ancestors who lived in caves. Even the alleged "whole grain" bakery products in most grocery stores are allowed to contain 49% refined white flour. Actually, most whole grain products are made by simply reconstituting white flour with bran and molasses for color.

As with refined sugar, the nutrients in flour are removed to make a product that is cheaper to produce and easier to store. This process does make a more handsome product, but also one that enhances corporate profits at the expense of the consumer's nutritional needs. We have been brainwashed to think that eggs and butter are the bad guys, when it is the toast and cereals at the breakfast table that are really harming us. White flour has virtually no meaningful nutrition. It has been enriched with folic acid and iron. It is very possible that the Ferris sulphate is harmful to many who will ingest it, such as men with coronary diseases and heart trouble. Essentially, white flour is like a mild shot of sugar and has more chance of adding to the fat load that the energy level of the one who consumes it. We discussed other challenges of wheat, gliadin and gluten earlier.

The "Beef" with Beef

I once worked in a butcher shop, and on another occasion I worked in the meat department of a supermarket. As a result, I know first hand how ground beef is made. All beef trimmings, even some from the floor—with a little flavorful sawdust—are saved for the grinder. I have seen ground beef made with nothing but fat and a bucket of blood added for color. I have seen display packages that have turned brown be repacked with a layer of pink freshly ground around the outside. The industry has a bundle of little tricks to enhance the appearance of meat and its water-weight.

The truth is, beef cattle are fattened in filth, housed in such close quarters that they must be given antibiotics to prevent them from infecting each other. They are slaughtered and butchered in that same filth. It is no surprise, then, to see the government report that the greater percentage of ground beef presented to the American consumer is contaminated with E. Coli and other bacteria. I am among those who are concerned about the energy the meat carries from the trauma of the slaughter.

The government's answer to this situation? Irradiation. Irradiation is the process of exposing food to high levels of radiation to reduce bacteria. The government claims that these energy waves affect only the bad micro-organisms. Officials say that the waves are not retained in the food. Why, then, does irradiation change the flavor of dairy products and soften the flesh of such fruits as peaches and nectarines? The reality is that we do not know what ill effects irradiation brings. It's too early to tell. We do know that irradiation causes mutations of DNA and changes the molecular structure of material exposed to it. Could this include a mutation of the vital amino acids in the protein we seek from meat?

Wouldn't it be safer to clean up or enlarge the holding pens where the cattle are fattened on estrogenic growth hormones? Safer, yes, but not as economical. So we decide to irradiate the meat instead. Or if you prefer the latest euphemism, you might say, "electronically pasteurize" the meat.

Today, we can fix infected meat products with a zapper equal to as many as a million chest x-rays. Then we can freeze it and microwave it. How good do you suppose those amino acids are? Radiation at any level can damage RNA and DNA. At the level of a million chest x-rays, meat or any other substance certainly undergoes mutation. And did I mention that irradiation takes place in a chamber with three foot thick concrete walls? How safe is that?

Perhaps the biggest problem of all is the big lie—irradiation doesn't keep us safe. Despite the continuous dosing of feed and dairy cattle with antibiotics, the cases of bacteria passed to humans through food are becoming more and more frequent. Many scientists warn that continued use of antibiotics provides an environment that encourages the mutation of bacteria. Apparently, we have reached that day of reckoning. Despite the use of irradiation, the number of cases of drug-resistant E. Coli are widespread. Deaths and serious illness are reported worldwide, especially numerous in Canada, the United States and Japan.

In January 2001, the Union of Concerned Scientists reported that 70% of nearly 25 million pounds of antibiotics are fed to healthy food animals yearly, 10.3 million to hogs, 10.5 million to chickens, and 3.7 million to cattle. It was unclear if the latter included dairy herds. The UCS believes that this overuse of antibiotics contributes to the growth of drug resistant bacteria. The group believes that the primary cause of drug resistance is the overuse of this class of drugs, and says that the massive non-therapeutic use of these antibiotics in food production has to be a major contributor to the problem.

Slaughter herds are fed growth hormones, too. A patch in the ear can add about $100 in weight to each head of cattle. A patch illegally placed on the rump will add about considerably more. Dairy cattle are given similar hormones to increase milk production. This practice has little or no regulation. It is up to each herdsman to determine the amount of these hormones that are to be used and how often.

We do not know exactly what the residual hormones do to the human body, but we do know that estrogen drives unwanted cell growth in the human body. A tumor is one form of unwanted cell growth. We may not know the impact these growth hormones have on human obesity in our lifetime, but there are legions of nutritionists and natural healers who believe that there is a direct connection between growth hormones used in food production and human obesity. If these hormones make one mammal increase in size and body fat, it is pretty clear what could happen to the mammal that consumes the product.

It is documented that an eight-year-old child who eats two fast food burgers will have a 25% hormone imbalance. There are some things taking place that could also be directly related to these female hormones. Men are balding younger. Male pattern balding at one time would begin around 35 or 40; today it begins for some in high school. We also have the "feminization" of the American male. This is under study by anthropologists, but it could well be a concern of nutritionists. Younger generations show less and less physical gender differences.

Another phenomenon is the number of girls who begin menses before age 10. This too is believed by many of us to be caused by the deluge of estrogens in the American diet and lifestyle. The only way to be sure your meat and dairy products are not filled with antibiotics and hormones it to buy organic. The organic label also gives assurance that the product has not been subjected to irradiation. However, careful shoppers will be glad to know that more and more meat and poultry products are coming to market that are hormone and antibiotic free and that are grass fed without being labeled organic. Meat and especially red meat are getting a bad name in some quarters. A food staple that has been with us since before the recorded word did not suddenly become a poison. It is not the meat, it is if the processing. Animals are supposed to eat grass. They do not have the digestive capabilities demanded for grains. Yes, grains fatten cattle for market, but not without serious challenges to the health of the animal and the consumer. It is worth noting that genetically modified organisms cannot be labeled organic. So far it is believed that some genetically modified farm raised fish are reaching the market. There is active research toward genetically modifying animals for food. There is a program in Germany that may be genetically modifying pigs with human genes in an effort to create a harvest of organs for human transplant. (Excuse me while it barf.)

It took a decade for the USDA to carry out the directions of the Congress in establishing standards for the organic label. It took years of testimony and debate to convince officials that organic food could not be raised in sewer sludge, could not be genetically modified, could not have chemical and antibiotic residue or other contaminants commonly present in conventionally produced food. Only a constant vigil has kept congress from eroding the organic standards by hiding riders and amendments in non-food legislation. Your Senator and Representative in the House are under powerful pressure from the food lobby to gut the organic regulations. Only continued grassroots pressure from consumers and voters can counter the sway of politics.

∽∽

Please! It Ain't Cheese!

It is fitting that the USDA listed processed cheese food last in its list of America's favorite foods because it incorporates all of the above, plus salt and refined oils. First of all we should address the long-standing rip off of the consumers and taxpayers. Milk farmers nationwide are paid for their milk based on the price from a little town in Wisconsin. Through powerful and generous lobbies, the industry uses legislation that was passed to stabilize milk prices during WWII to inflate prices for dairy products today.

The government buys the surplus milk to create an artificial shortage. This milk is converted to powdered milk and cheese food. That stuff that is called cheddar cheese that falls off the back of trucks and appears in senior centers is not real cheese. Real cheese costs at least three times more than a true market would support. We are paying to support an industry that is protected by the government. Our reward is cheese at more than ten dollars a pound that would probably cost three dollars in a true market. We are paying on both ends, and the small or independent farmer is squeezed more than the udders of the cows he relies on to make his living.

So, enter processed cheese food. "American Cheese." What is it made from? Refined oils, white flour, artificial coloring, artificial flavors, chemical binders, chemical preservatives, and some milk, usually bought from the government's stores of powdered milk. The government pays a fair price for it, pays a political pork barrel price to store it, and then sells it cheap to dairy processors. It ain't fair, and it ain't cheese.

Ever Wonder Why It Is Called Junk Food?

So-called junk food in the standard American Diet tends to incorporate all of the above so-called fast food items. The growth of the convenience or drive-thru food industry in America corresponds to the growth of diet-related diseases, according to many scientists. The total blame does not rest solely on the fast food restaurants, but they are the ones who developed the recipes for our pop food culture. They studied our weak and indulgent tongue sensations and set about to please us. School lunch programs, cafeterias and food processors followed their lead. The result is a super-sized mentality and a diet that panders to our tongue sensations or "mouth feel" with only a minuscule of concern for nutrition. If that much!

Scientists at SUNY Buffalo analyzed the effects of a super-sized breakfast from McDonalds. They found increased inflammation in the veins and a host of other negatives within hours of eating the McMuffin with a double order of hash browns. Surprise! It was not the eggs and sausage that caused the problems. The problems were caused by the white flour bun, the components of the artificial cheese and the oils used to cook the hash browns.

So, how about a cheeseburger on a fluffy white flour bun? How about some macaroni and cheese from the microwave? Washed down with a diet soda? Does it still sound as good as ever?

A Sprinkle of Salt

Many manufactured foods have a high salt content. The American Heart Association recommends that healthy adults consume no more than 2400 milligrams of sodium daily. This is equivalent to about 1 ¼ teaspoon of table salt. But as you may have guessed, most of us consume much more. In fact, we consume three times the recommended amount every day. While we do not need such an abundance of sodium, it is true that we do need some salt.

I do not think we need salt that is dug from the earth, however. A modest amount of natural sea salt is a better nutritional component. We found out in the latter 1930s that people needed more iodine in their salt. When we were switched from sea salt to mined salt, the lack of natural iodine led to goiters. When the thyroid gland does not get enough iodine, it becomes enlarged. The increased size allows it to produce the hormones the body needs for balance with less nutrition. There was an epidemic of goiters from the iodine deficiency created by the use of salt from mines. So did we go back to sea salt? No. We created a new industry—mining iodine to reconstitute the salt from other mines.

But you see, sea salt has a natural amount of iodine already contained within it. The saline of our bodies should be the same as seawater. However God went about creating us, seawater was surely involved. It makes sense to me that our bodies would get along better with the real thing than a man-manipulated substitute. The need for salt is without dispute. But the fact remains that too much salt can crowd out much needed calcium, our most plentiful body mineral. Also, too much salt reduces our electrolyte activity.

Salt is sodium chloride. Sodium molecules have a positive electrical charge, and chloride has a negative charge. Potassium with a positive charge works between the sodium and the chloride to cause movement. This movement is necessary for nutrients to get into our cells and for toxins to get out. It also influences bowel contractions that control the transit time for our waste matter. The ratio of potassium over sodium chloride salt should be 5:1. For many who think they are using too much salt, it is very possible that they simply do not have sufficient potassium in their daily diet.

A Word About Oils

The edible oil industry is a major part of the agricultural economy of our country. At one time it was believed that inexpensive vegetable oil such as corn would become a renewable energy source. The Diesel engine was developed to run on vegetable oil. It was believed that vegetable oil would power our cars, trucks and trains. More important, it would fuel the big Diesel engines that turn the generators in our electric power plants. Perhaps, vegetable oil was a threat to the infrastructure of the more established petroleum industry. That is how vegetable oil became a food.

Anybody who tells you that margarine is better than butter is either ignorant or a mouth for hire, or both. The coagulants used to make oils solid at room temperature also make them solid in your body. There is a strong movement within the scientific community (among those who do not work for food manufacturers) to support warning labels for margarine and shortening. Warning labels have not been required, but some communities have demanded a reduction or elimination of trans fats.

The reason? These fats are made of hydrogenated oils. Hydrogenated oils are the oils that can clog the arteries. There are some spreads on the market which contain a concentration of plant ester compounds that can improve high cholesterol readings, but margarine is still margarine—even with some good stuff added. Preliminary studies show that the same spreads claiming to improve cholesterol results may also reduce body stores of a very important nutrient, Vitamin A.

Refined oils are much like other refined foods; they are distorted. Their molecules have been changed, and they are non-nutritive. Perhaps worse, these refined oils can bond with our good oils—our essential fatty acids—to render them worthless. We need our Omega

3 and Omega 6 oils, unrefined, everyday. The IQ of American young-sters is decreasing a little more every year. Many believe that the re-fined oils are negating the small amount of essential fatty acids that remain in the diet.

Because of the way they are processed, refined oils are an un-desirable non-nutrient. Most vegetable oils have a short lifespan and quickly turn rancid. This is why they are refined. Here are some of the steps vegetable oils undergo when being refined: First, they are treated with chemicals similar to those used to make drain cleaners and glass degreasers. Then they are bleached. By now they are clear, but they stink. The smell is eliminated by boiling. If the heat used to expel it and the chemicals used to clarify it do not make refined oils an undesirable food, then the boiling will finish the job. Although these oils have a nice appearance in their clear plastic bottles on the grocery store shelf, they are really just fat-producing non-nutrients. They are trans fatty acids. Trans fatty acids are produced when most vegetable oils are heated above 220 degrees F. Partial hydrogenation requires heat in excess of 500 degrees F.

If you would like to know more about oil, I suggest you read *"Fats That Heal, Fats That Kill"* by Udo Erasmus. He has a brilliant ex-planation of the role played in our health by the essential fatty acids, the fats that heal. We need the essential fatty acids to produce good brain cells and nourish the mind. They are also important for an ac-tive adrenal system and a responsive immune system.

Heat distorts most oils. The oil becomes a trans fatty coagu-lant—similar to those fats used to make margarine. One reason the Mediterranean diet does not work for Americans is because of the way we use oil. We like to sauté our vegetables in lots of oil. After all, we were told that using lots of olive oil is good for us. But we should be cooking like a Mediterranean—steam or poach the vegetables and then pour on generous amounts of olive oil. Or sauté with a little sat-urated fat.

There is a definite link between refined oils and high meat consumption with inflammatory conditions and joint pain. AA, ara-chidonic acid, is a valuable long chain polyunsaturated fatty acid in balanced amounts. Too much of a good thing, again, is not a good thing. The excess AA thrown into the body by these refined oils easily converts to eicosanoids such as series 2 prostaglandins with a double bond side chain. This imbalance leads to inflammation and joint pain. This condition can contribute to <u>any</u> inflammatory disease. At this point the worthless refined oils and the excess AA overwhelm the vital Omega 3 fatty acids. Under normal conditions the Omega 3 will transfer to eicosapentaenoic acid (EPA) and to DHA, docosohexaenoic acid. EPA controls prostaglandin 2 to reduce inflammation and joint pain. DHA is our most vital daily nutrient for a healthy brain and good cognitive function.

Can these refined oils contribute to dementia and arthritis? Yes. They also can accelerate the aging process throughout the body. Good and active metabolism depends on Omega 3 essential fatty acid. Yes, a deficiency can contribute to weight gain and obesity. Consumption of trans fatty acids that diminish the Omega 3 can cause the deficiency that leads to weight gain. They also defy digestion and can be stored in their fatty state.

As these trans fatty acids enter the body, they slide out of the liver into the blood stream where they contribute to triglycerides, cholesterol and other lipids. The body's immune system perceives trans fatty acids to be pathogens. As the immune system goes after these "perceived-pathogens" it creates an inflammatory condition. This inflammation contributes to any number of conditions including heart disease, cancer, arthritis, Alzheimer's and dementia or others including compromised metabolism and obesity.

We can learn a valuable lesson about vegetable oil from cattle ranchers. In the 1940s ranchers tried to fatten cattle with inexpensive coconut oil. It did not work. The animals did not gain weight, even when their caloric input was increased. They tried giving them a thyroid suppressant to slow down their metabolism. It worked, but it was too toxic with harsh side effects. They tried soy and corn oils. The found that the soy would suppress the thyroid and that the cattle gained weight with less food. However, corn oil is known to suppress the immune system. They tried the new wonder drugs, the antibiotics that had just been discovered. Corn and soy to fatten the cattle with the help of a sub therapeutic dose of antibiotics continues to be the standard of the industry to the present day. One other addition has been put into use today, the estrogen growth hormones.

Ditch the Junk Food

Scientists in Saudi Arabia and Scotland have established a link between the rise of junk food establishments and the rise in the number of youngsters being treated for asthma and allergies. In France Jose Bove, the sheep farmer who trashed a fast food establishment in protest of the spread of junk food, spent time in jail. Even so, he says he is proud to have spoken up for nutrition. Studies in the UK and at Harvard Medical School have found that teens who eat a predominately junk-food diet have the veins of a person in his or her 40s. These young people have all the markers for future heart disease and diabetes.

Dr. Gerald Bernstein, a past president of the American Diabetes Association and an endocrinologist with Beth Israel Medical Center in New York City, fears the number of cases of adult-onset diabetes, or Type 2 diabetes will nearly double in the next 20 years. He and others warned that adult-onset diabetes is reaching epidemic proportions, especially among the young. Normally this disease strikes people over 50 years of age. In the late summer of 2000, however, research showed that an estimated 50% of those coming down with adult-onset diabetes were children between 9 and 19! The Centers for Disease Control in Atlanta issued a report showing a 70% increase in the number of people between 30 and 39 with adult onset diabetes, which represents a 40% increase in individuals between 40 and 49 years of age, and an increase of 31% in the over 50 group. The rise in obesity is seen as a factor spurring the rise in diabetes cases.

I am compelled to include some developments from the summer of 2005 that included the American Diabetic Association. The chief medical and scientific officer of the ADA has proclaimed that, "There is no evidence that sugar itself has anything to do with diabetes." Ignoring years of scientific study and evidence, Richard Kahn asked, "Where is the evidence?"

His proclamation came a few weeks before the ADA announced a three-year multi-million dollar alliance with Cadbury Schweppes. The company is a major producer of candy and the third largest maker of sodas and other beverages. I suppose that a flood being a condition that involves a body of water exceeding its normal containment has nothing to do with rain. And booze has nothing to do with alcoholism.

A few weeks later Andrew Briscoe, President of the Sugar Association, told the Alliance convention in Sun Valley that, "There is no link between sugar and obesity," and that "every major, comprehensive review of the total body of scientific literature continues to exonerate sugar intake as a causative factor in any lifestyle disease, including obesity."

Briscoe noted that sugar consumption is actually down from 102 pounds per person in 1972 to an estimated 63 pounds per person today. *(This does not mean that people are watching their sugar intake. The figure is down because since 1972 High Fructose Corn Syrup has replaced sugar as the commercial sweetener of choice.)* "Sugar is not part of the obesity issue," Briscoe said. "We believe in calories in and calories out."

In the same time frame and in response to dozens of school districts removing all soda dispensers, The American Beverage Association announced a compromise to keep the beverage machines in the lucrative locations on school property. At the meeting of the National Conference of State Legislators in Seattle, the organization's CEO, Susan Neely, announced unanimous approval by the ABA board for a set of guidelines that will eliminate sodas from all but half the dispensers in high schools. In elementary schools only water and 100% juices will be dispensed. In middle schools only lower calorie beverages will be offered. At high schools no more than half of the beverages offered will be sodas. (Note that sports drinks, tea and other popular beverages can contain as much HFCS as sodas.) The ABA is asking school districts and beverage distributors to follow these new guidelines. Neely said, "Childhood obesity is a serious problem in the U.S., and the responsibility of a common-sense solution is shared by our industry."

Too much food and super-sized portions are a major part of our problem. Dr. Marion Nestle who is director of the Department of Nutrition and Food Sciences at New York University points out that while most Americans need about 2,000 calories per day, the food industry is producing 3,800 calories for every person. Dr. Nestle thinks this competition among food producers forces them to over promote consumption especially among children. This pressure to eat more and more often is causing obesity and health problems.

The big gulp, super-size mentality is made worse by a lack of physical activity. Exercise uses calories and burns off some of the glucose clogging the cells, the liver and the body in general. It is easy to understand that using up some of the excess glucose will make it easier for the pancreas to deliver the insulin and the cells to use it. As they say, this is not rocket science; it is simple common sense. If we eat more than we use, we make fat. If we keep eating fat producing foods we will keep producing fat.

Our health problems will continue to increase until we get back to growing and eating real food—food that has not tricked Mother Nature into some kind of eye pleasing empty harvest. Food that has not been processed until the meager nutrition is lost. Food that is cooked with modest heat which enhances its ability to nourish. Food that feeds us, rather than food that is robbing us of our vitality, our energy and our health.

We have discussed the problems that tongue sensations, America's favorite foods, salt, and oils bring, and here is the conclusion we must draw: The way we eat is making us sick and fat. The medicine we have to take for the sickness is killing us. We are the human race, the survivors. Maybe it is time to think about some changes. For one thing, we should ask why the same government agency that oversees the foods that make us sick also oversees the medical industry that is supposed to cure us. Einstein said, "The answers to problems do not come from the same state of consciousness that created them". We owe it to ourselves to actively pursue answers to all our health and nutrition questions. It is imperative if we want to improve our diets and health.

The Harvard Medical School came up with a novel idea to improve eating habits—family dinners. Their study concludes that teens who have dinner with their families are more likely to eat good vegetables than junk food.

Family dinners not only nourish our bodies, but they also nourish our relationships and our souls. I believe that the kitchen stove is the modern campfire and that we should all gather around at the end of every day. We should participate in the preparation and presentation of the meal. It deserves candles and soft music—no TV or cell phones. We should come to the table with ground rules: Pick no fights. This is no time for reprimands. Anything that does not show love and appreciation for one another has to wait. Mealtime is family time for spiritual and love renewal. We all need that; we all crave that. These are hungers we can feed. It is our food that replenishes the elements of our bodies that came out of the Earth, yes Mother Earth.

Startling Statistics

Consider this. Despite a call from the World Health Organization for countries to limit allowable sugar content to no more than 10%, the Bush administration decided to continue the policy of the Clinton White House and allow 25% sugar. Most sodas, by the way, are closer to 1/3 sugar or high fructose corn syrup.

Let's look at what the government has issued as a guideline for food intake: Sugar and other sweeteners–25%. The latest USDA modified recommendation calls for grains at 50%.

Any way one might want look at these guidelines they will still come to 75% fat-making carbohydrate, in the standard American diet. The remaining 25% will probably come from degenerative vegetable oils with trans fatty acids and grain fed meat and dairy. All of which contribute to fat making and poor metabolism.

Now, is it clear why illness and obesity prevail in our country? Is it clear why diet programs and exercise are not reducing our waistlines? We are gorged with fat-making foods that starve us for the essential nutrition our bodies need to be healthy and in balance.

90% of the average family food budget goes for processed food. My daughter looked in our pantry one day during a visit and declared, "There is nothing in here but ingredients." I was impressed by her perception, and I hope she was impressed by our resolve to give our bodies the elements from the Earth needed to keep us in health and balance.

I know that I have painted a depressing picture of the state of our food delivery system, but it is accurate and well researched. I have tried to lay the facts bare for you to draw your own conclusions. I may have depressed you. That was certainly not a goal. If anything I hope I have inspired you to take control of your life and make your own decisions without being led down the rosy path by statements and recommendations that do not serve your best interest. In Europe consumers have dominated the marketplace. They have managed to keep most of the toxic products off the shelves of their stores. They did not do it at the ballot box. They did it where they found more power–the cash register. If American consumers simply ignore or boycott products, those products will soon disappear. Retailers want to sell their inventory, and they will stock the inventory that you buy. Let them know what you want and watch them scramble for your business.

Swing That Revolving Door One More Time

BPA, Bisphenol A, is a controversial substance in the news of late. It is in plastics used for baby bottles, plastic wrap and it is created often in the packaging and canning process. Here is what scientists are saying about BPA: *Journal of the American Medical Association,* reports that it is linked to cardiovascular disease and diabetes. The National Toxicology Program concluded that there is "some concern" that fetuses, babies and children were in danger because of BPA. Some scientists suspect that exposure early in life disrupts hormones and alters genes, programming genes for breast and prostate cancer later in life, premature female puberty, ADD and other reproductive and neurological disorders.

Dr. Martin Philbert of the FDA approved BPA as safe according to industry standards. By the way, Philbert is founder and co-director of University of Michigan Risk Science Center. A medical supply manufacturer, by the name of Charles Gelman, decides out of the goodness of his heart to give $5 million dollars to the research center. His donation is 50 times the annual budget of the research center. Mind you this is the same manufacturer that is saying that Bisphenol A is safe.

The Dairy Education Board has traced the pattern of events that has given the green light so many Monsanto proposals. Prior to being the Supreme Court Judge who put George Bush in office, Clarence Thomas was Monsanto's lawyer. The U.S. Secretary of Agriculture (Anne Veneman) was on the Board of Directors of Monsanto's Calgene Corporation. The Secretary of Defense (Donald Rumsfeld) was on the Board of Directors of Monsanto's Searle pharmaceuticals. The U.S. Secretary of Health, Tommy Thompson, received $50,000 in donations from Monsanto during his winning campaign for Wisconsin's governor. The two congressmen receiving the most donations from Monsanto during the last election were Larry Combest (Chairman of the House Agricultural Committee) and Attorney General John Ashcroft.

The connection has become expected and is so common that nobody bothers to keep it a secret. It is right out there in our face every day.

The Final Mutilation

After all our food goes through on the vine, after all it goes through after harvest including shipment of an average 1,500 miles for each item, the final mutilation comes at home when we pop it into the microwave. One of the dumbest things I have seen lately is a plastic bag of organic spinach with instructions to cook it in the bag in the microwave. Why bother with organic when it is going to be exposed to the radiation that changes its molecular structure in a plastic bag that will leech it full of phthalates and Bisphenol A? It is amazing that the microwave has become a central convenience item in the American home to be used by health conscious people who are buying quality food at premium prices only to mutilate it for convenience

The microwave oven was invented in Nazi Germany. The Germans had their eyes on Russia and knew the history of how the Russian geography had beaten back the conquering hordes on several occasions throughout history. The microwave was to be used to keep warm food available for the marching army across the frozen tundra of Russia on the road to Moscow. Well as it turned out the Russians were in Berlin before the Germans could carry out their plans. The Russians would end up in possession of the microwave oven and related technology. After a few tests and scientific examinations the Russian abandoned the microwave and actually banned production of more. It was the Swiss who did the conclusive studies on the microwave and they banned it. Leave it to the Americans to sell it to their own people.

The Swiss found that the heat is caused by friction. The radiation causes the atoms in the molecules to vibrate so rapidly and fiercely that they get hot from the friction. That is why the food from a microwave has hot spots and cold spots causing one to wait until the hot spots can convey the heat to the cold spots before eating it. In the process the atoms vibrate with such force that they crash through the wall of their molecule and bombard another molecule. This changes the structure of the food and creates what it called *radiotrons*. It is a substance that has never existed before in nature, and it is not the same thing that it was when it went into the micro-mutilation machine. It is like plastic. Try it with a slice of bread. In thirty seconds you have created a rubbery substance that is too tough to chew. That is the story on the microwave.

I believe that food from the microwave has lost some or most of its nutritional value. Enzymes, amino acids, bioflavonoids and other beneficial components are mutilated. The user has turned a fresh vegetable into a junk, empty-calorie food.

‿‿

The Spiritual Power to Lose It

If you are hoping this book will put you on the cover of the *Sports Illustrated* swimsuit issue, you might be disappointed. This book does not promise to turn you into a super model, male or female. My goal is to show you why you may have lost control of your waistline and to help you regain control. It is also my goal to help you understand that you are a very special individual. If you are not happy with your appearance and if your weight is casting a shadow over your self-esteem, this book is for you. If you have issues with yourself other than weight you may also find this book helpful in achieving greater health and focus.

Each of us has a special place in the fabric of the Universe. If we are not all or everything we should be, or if we do not have self-love and self-respect, the whole world is missing something very special. You and me. We all need each other. If I let myself go and drift into a condition that does not allow me to walk with pride and present myself with confidence, I am not only letting myself down, I am letting you down. If you are not capable of mustering the courage to present your excellence to the world, both of us are missing your unique contribution. It has been said that the world can be changed in a heartbeat; certainly we have the power to change our own personal world. I believe if we change the conditions within us and around us, we have done our part in changing the world.

Each of us has the power to make the most of what we have to work with. Beauty is not found in the shape of our body; it is in the excellence and love of our spirit. The world sees us as we present ourselves. If we want to change the way the world sees us, we must change the way we see ourselves.

Your Own Uniqueness

You will gain respect in your journey that is in direct proportion to the respect you have for yourself. The first step in having control of your body, is accepting it the way it came into the world. No amount of dieting, starvation, surgery or exercise can turn a Ford into a Chevy. Your individual journey is to the realization of what God intended when you were conceived. Whatever that might be is beautiful, necessary and worthy.

You must realize that you are unique and that the world needs you the way you came into it. The world needs the "you" that may be hiding in the shadows of your mind and flesh because you have decided that you don't measure up to the modern conception of "pop beauty." Do you realize that hiding behind the shadows of some super-model's mind there may be a person wishing they could have your gifts?

We are diverse in everything that we are. Every generation and culture has its conception of what pretty people are supposed to look like. It is not what you look like that is important; it is what you really are, inside and out, that the world is waiting to see unfold.

Looking like something does not make it so. You do not need to make a new body to be what you are supposed to be. However, if your body does not represent you the way you want to present yourself to the world, you also have the power to change it. All the power you need for this journey is already inside you. My goals with this book are to challenge you to look inside yourself for answers to your problems—and for control of your life. These answers do not come from the outside.

Energy as Catalyst

Modern physics teaches us that energy needs an attractor. It is a force that guides the energetics of change. As creatures of habit we spend much, sometimes all, of our lives stuck in a pattern of habits that keep us in the same old circles of activity—or inactivity. Our concept of self in psychiatry is known as the ego. The ego can be nothing more than a series of habits that guide our activity and block our growth spiritually and physically. We need an attractor to guide our change and growth; otherwise we are stuck in the ruts of old habits.

Most of our ego is shaped by comments about us from people around us in our formative years. We are bombarded with old sayings that demoralize and deflate us. Even from the lips of our loved ones come thousands of years of negative sayings that shape our concept of ourselves, or our ego. This is hard to shake.

Many times the abuses are not limited to verbal assaults. How many women and men do you know that have a hard time appreciating themselves and honoring themselves because they were hurt so deeply by sexual or physical abuses. We probably have no idea how many of the people we come in contact with regularly whose lives are shaped by these kinds of events. Many never get past the depression and gnawing anger that come from these experiences. Whatever the reason for these emotional extremes, they can be an abyss with no foreseeable way out.

Faith is energy. Faith is the energy that can be the catalyst that changes our lives. Science teaches us that all matter is really energy. After molecules come the atoms. When we take the atom apart, the sub-particles vanish leaving only the energetic vibrations.

Even things we perceive as solid matter are only energy with a form of vibrating substance. When we are focused on the present moment, our faith is all powerful. That is when the mustard seed of faith moves a mountain. Faith is energy lacking form, or the evidence of things not yet seen. Faith is an energy that has not yet taken substantive form in your life, but it **will** at some point.

Forgiveness and Release?

Forgiveness cannot be achieved in anger. In time, when our wounds are less tender, we might understand more about the behavior that harmed us. We may or may not be able to forgive. While forgiveness may be too much to ask or expect, releasing our anger is necessary for self-preservation. When we release our anger and resentments, it is an act of tenderness for ourselves separate from forgiveness. So, whether or not we are able to forgive in time, learning to let go is essential for health and certainly for happiness today. It is difficult to realize that being victimized does not give us the power of condemnation or the right to punish for vengeance or to carry out what we perceive to be justice. We all pay for what we do. It comes back to us many fold. This is a natural law as vivid and certain as the law of gravity. Those who have harmed us have a destiny with a justice greater than what we would design for them. We help ourselves most by having faith in that greater justice. Only when we let go of the anger can we energize our own healing. The anger keeps us a victim, and the image of a victim lessens our concept of self. Eventually this can lead to physical illness. More immediately, anger distorts our self-image. It is our self-image, or ego, that can distort and determine the shape of our body. Whatever has happened to us, anger may do more harm to us than the event. We must use our faith and learn to let go.

Smokers have to reshape their self-image to see themselves as non-smokers before they are comfortable with giving up a habit they know is harmful to their bodies. Similarly, losing weight depends on being able to find a comfortable image of yourself as a thinner you. This may involve letting go of anger and memories of painful events. When the ego is entwined with anger or other damaging emotions, you are not free to experience change.

I firmly believe that changes in our behavior must begin at the spiritual level. Many programs designed to help people overcome damaging habits work because they take the person to a spiritual level of consciousness. If we are to make changes in our lives we must first change the ego, or visual concept we hold of ourselves.

Addressing the Ego

It is not easy to address the ego. Even things in our life that we know are harmful and damaging to us can be hard to give up. We continue abusive habits or stay in bad relationships because we are not prepared to fill the empty space the change would leave in our perception of ourselves. We drift into a zone of relative comfort as we adapt to a life that accommodates harmful habits and a chaotic environment.

Without addressing the ego, some attempts at change initially fail. For example, many people stop smoking, only to end up smoking more than ever when they revert back to their favorite habit. Many people can lose weight, but end up packing on more pounds when they revert. Sadly, many people ruin their health with so-call yoyo diets–which bring short-term weight loss but long term weight gains. Weight fluctuations can be dangerous. In all of these cases, it is highly likely that the individuals were reverting to an image of themselves that had not changed. They lost weight in their bodies, or stopped smoking, but still thought of themselves as a heavy person or as a smoker. The old image was the attractor that led them back to the old life. We must again use our faith. We must know that what will fill the voids of our being when we give up negative habits, will be enriching to our lives in every way. What comes to us in faith is always better than what we can plan, and certainly better than what might befall us from unfocused chaos.

When I counsel with people I urge them to project an image of themselves in faith. Remember, faith is energy as much as any other vibration; it simply has not taken physical or solid form yet. Make the attractor of your energy a projection in faith. Let it be an affirmation. "Thank You for making me the beautiful and unique person that I am." This image will be the attractor of the energy of change in your body and your life. It will pull you toward what God intends you to be. Yes, all things do really work together for those that love the Lord, or otherwise affirm their faith.

Gaining Control
by Re-Imagining

I believe that surrender is control. As long as we try to create our journey from an ego or perception of self that was shaped by chaotic sources outside us, we are doomed to a life of bad habits. The older we get the deeper the ruts of the behavior pattern. We seem to go around in the same old circles making the same old mistakes and experiencing the same sense of failure. When we surrender to God's intention for us, we gain control of our lives.

At first "through a glass darkly" you can behold your new image. You may not be able to visualize the clear image of yourself. How could you? You do not know this person yet. As the attractor guides your journey in faith, the energy of your changes will put this person in clearer perspective. You will get out of the ruts of old habits. You will shape a new image in the true likeness of God's intention.

The most courageous thing we do in life is not heroics in a tragedy; it is taking the first steps on the journey to self. "What if we do not like what we find? What if I am not nice, not worthy, not beautiful?" I challenge you to find the courage to go on the inward journey to self. I also promise you that if you persist on this journey, you will like what you find. You will like yourself.

Vast fortunes have been made by those who promise easy solutions to achieve changes in body image. Many claim to have the magic pill that will take off the pounds while you sleep, and they promise you do not have to change your lifestyle. How many people do you know who are constantly sending away for the latest diet pill or diet plan? In the time you have known them, have they gained control of their weight? I like to say, "There are no magic chants, there are no magic potions and there are no gurus." The magic and the guidance are inside you.

Every cell of your body holds the intelligence of Creation. Do not be afraid to think with your heart and your gut instincts. Both are smarter than the brain. If you are not happy with your body, you have the power to make changes. Once you realize that the basic package is uniquely you and nobody else, you are ready to make the most of it. We are all beautiful when we show the world our inner excellence. We make ourselves grotesque when we lack the courage and faith to be exactly the person our genetic and spiritual heritage determined for us. With courage and faith we find God's intention for us.

You may find that food has served a purpose for you as a kind of comfort or excuse to avoid the reality of the true self. If this is the case, focus on the present; release the past, and know that the best preparation for tomorrow is to live this moment with pride, passion and zeal. You do not have to be ashamed of the way you look. The power for change is within you. All you have to do is believe and make healthy lifestyle changes and food choices–little by little. The world is waiting to meet the true you.

☙❧

Stepping Forward:
Sculpting the Real You

You can visually sculpt your body by claiming the shape it is supposed to have in faith. Your mind and your spirit will make the changes as you take away the foods that have distorted it. The "eat all you want" diet plan that I present in this book allows you to eat all you want of the right foods. At the same time it eliminates those foods that are responsible for the conditions that are making you uncomfortable.

Please, do not think in terms of what you have to give up. Be open to the discovery of all the foods that may not be part of your life at this time. Much of what you will be asked to limit will be temporary. Once you reach your desired weight, you can put many of these items back into your daily diet. There are some things you should never touch again, but you will be so empowered by pride and confidence in your weight loss that you will no longer desire those things that might stall your progress.

Step forward in faith, free from the shadows of the past and "free from the fears of tomorrow."

Change is constant because energy has constant vibration. Energy needs an attractor. The change, or energy, that defines our journey in life also needs an attractor. Without an attractor our energy is spent in chaotic habits, good and bad. When we affirm in faith an image of God's intention for us we create the attractor for the energy of change in our journey that will lead us to our true self.

There are a few things that you must start or continue doing each day to gain control of your weight and reach your life goals in general. They are not complicated and they do not require a lot of time or sacrifice. Perhaps, just a little discipline to get started will be necessary.

Spiritual Renewal

Although I am an ordained minister, I do not consider it my role in this context to tell you how to be spiritual or to suggest one ritual or religion over another. We are as unique in our spirituality as we are in all other aspects of our lives.

I do suggest that you return to your roots if you are not currently engaged in active spiritual renewal. I really do not believe that we have to embrace rituals from another culture or belief system to become more spiritual. Whatever your faith or belief system, make time several times each day to connect your consciousness to your faith. This keeps us centered, and it is necessary for good energy flow through our bodies.

I often tell people not to leave home and go into the world until they have touched the quiet peace of their inner faith. Stay in touch with it at all times. It has a way of keeping things in perspective. There is nothing more powerful for reducing stress than inner peace.

Spiritual renewal also helps us let go of the emotions that can challenge our health and wellbeing. Anger, for example, leads to stress on the heart, the liver and the immune system. It adds to the stress hormones that trigger the metabolism that causes girth weight gain. Dr John Swartzberg, of the University of California at Berkley, writing in the *Wellness Letter* suggests meditation and other means as a way of releasing anger before it begins to harm the body.

Anger also can increase the abuse of tobacco, alcohol and other substances—including food and the incidence of eating disorders. No matter what has happened to you to make you angry, you should know that the anger is doing far more harm to your body and your life than the event. The only person you harm with your anger is yourself. Letting go frees us from the bonds of anger. If you have an eating disorder, it may be tied to anger or some other emotion from a traumatic event that still haunts you. This also keeps you focused on the past and denies you the power of the present.

Change in human behavior originates at a spiritual level. Change requires energy, and energy requires an attractor. As we mentioned earlier, without an attractor we remain victims of our habits. I want to teach you a simple exercise for helping you to focus on the present moment.

Sit in a quiet place. Close your eyes and roll them toward the top of your head. Inhale as deeply as possible through your nose and exhale completely through your mouth. Do this three or four times, or until you feel meditative. Hold the last inhaled breath briefly. Gather all your thoughts and as you exhale through your mouth, let your brain go blank. When you open your eyes, it will be the beginning of your life. All that really matters is the moment at hand.

While you are focused on the present your faith is most powerful. At this time make an affirmation of faith as your attractor. Affirm a commitment to whatever God intended for you at the moment of your conception. Know that it is whole and beautiful. Know that it is a better plan than anything you might create. It is better than any goal you may set for yourself. With this attractor, the energy of your life will cause the changes, and you will grow into the person God intended. This is Divine order. Personal goals and other plans are chaos.

You will be guided by faith from this moment forward. I do not want you to set a goal for how many pounds you would like to lose. Simply follow the diet restrictions that will reduce the fat-making food and you will find your natural self.

As you prepare for this change remember, it is not about a scale or a target weight. It is about the fulfillment of your journey to self.

∽∽

Deep Breathing

Deep breathing is very important, in addition to the exercise above. It helps us to have spiritual focus and to focus on the present moment. It also fills our lungs with oxygen which is very energizing. Deep breathing improves digestion and elimination; it also helps produce B vitamins. Take a moment for a few deep breaths several times a day. You will be surprised what it can do for you.

Rest

The average American is sleep deprived almost every day. We all tend to need different amounts of sleep. Between late night TV and getting a jump on traffic the next morning, by the end of the week we have lost enough sleep to equal a full night of rest. We are on the go seven days a week with only six nights of sleep. Over time, this can cause deep trouble for our metabolism and our immune system.

It is important to sleep in darkness. Melatonin, serotonin and other important hormones are made while we sleep in the **darkness**. Night lights and other forms of light can keep us from making these important hormones. People who work at night and sleep during the day should wear a mask or otherwise make sure they experience total darkness while sleeping. Many people drift into insomnia because of a deficiency of serotonin and melatonin. They cannot sleep because they were not asleep in darkness long enough to make the hormones needed for sound sleep. Catch 22? Rest is also a shield against stress.

Water

Dehydration may be a bigger problem in America than obesity, it is just less obvious. Dehydration among older people is evident with a visit to almost any nursing home. My observation has been that many are being medicated for conditions that would be eliminated with adequate hydration. One of the major problems is the popular belief that any liquid will hydrate the body. This is not true. If we consume a liquid such as fruit juice that must be digested, we must surrender water to support the digestion. We can drink juice all day and it can lead to dehydration without adequate intake of pure water.

We also surrender water every time we exhale. This moistens our breath to help it carry toxins from the body. This moisture is also necessary to maintain the integrity of our nasal membranes. They become dry, and sinus conditions can develop without adequate water intake. In this diet plan you will be asked to consume 8 ounces of pure water for every 20 pounds of body weight. Many people retain water because they do not consume enough to flush their kidneys. This forces the body to dilute and store toxins, which leads to high blood pressure and swelling, especially around the ankles. The solution to water retention for many people is drinking more water.

Essential Nutrition

Every day we need substances that cannot be synthesized in the body. They are vitamins that the body cannot produce and minerals that must come from the earth. Two other groups of essential nutrients are fatty acids and amino acids. The fatty acids are Omega 3 and Omega 6. While the body can make many amino acids, endless combinations of them in fact, it cannot make the eight essential amino acids. These eight must be in our diet daily if we are to have balance and health. In fact, if we are missing any one of these essential nutrients in our diet, eventually that deficiency will present symptoms of one or more diseases. Numerous diseases are caused by a deficiency of one or more essential nutrients.

The Simple Plan

I suggest in this diet plan that you take supplements that will provide the essential nutrients. You have probably heard that it is better to get your vitamins and minerals from your food. I agree that it would be better to get your vitamins and minerals from food. At the same time, I would like to meet one person who really does get their essential nutrition solely from food, and I would like to know where they get the food that contains that much nutrition.

For the most part the minerals are not in the soil and the food does not ripen sufficiently to produce the vitamins and other nutrients needed to achieve the goal of complete nutrition. There are probably places on earth where sustainable agriculture is practiced and where people go to the village marketplace every morning to get their food for the day. That is not the experience of most Americans, however. Most of us shop every seven to ten days, and the food we buy is rarely harvested "this morning for consumption today." Until we can have access to freshly harvested food, we need supplements. One way of reducing hunger is by making sure your body is not asking for more food trying to satisfy its need for daily essential nutrition. As I outline this plan, please do not feel you are losing ALL of your favorite foods. Actually, many of them you will be able to have again when you have reached your desired weight. In the earlier pages we discussed the reasons for obesity and the foods that are associated with unwanted weight gain. This diet plan is simple in that it eliminates the foods that have been making more glucose and subsequent fat than you have been able to burn off, even with exercise.

Rule One–No sugar, HFCS, honey, syrup or other sweetener. This includes chemical artificial sweeteners such as sucralose (Splenda) or aspartame. (Stevia is allowed.)

The two main items we are going to eliminate or limit are sugars in all forms and grains. As we pointed our earlier, if we consume foods that are 25% sugar and follow the USDA guidelines to consume a diet that is 50% grain, it is a 75% fat-producing diet.

Eliminate Sugar, High Fructose Corn Syrup and other sweeteners. For many people, this will remove 25% of the fat producing foods from the diet. This will include soda, sports drinks, flavored fruit waters and even fruit juices. Fruit juice is filled with unbound fructose and can contribute to obesity. This one may be difficult, but it helps you keep a good relationship with pure water.

Rule Two–Only one serving per day of whole grain-(not wheat).

Remember how they fatten cattle for market? They pen them up and feed them grains. If you eliminate grains, especially refined grains, from your diet you have removed half of the cause of your weight gain. The USDA is calling for half of one's daily calories from grains. Wheat, corn, rye, oats, barley, rice and other foods are in the grain category. While the bran or insoluble fiber from whole grains is important for health, the end of the digestive process for grains remains, simple sugar. Simple sugar equals glucose–equals fat. If half your calories are from gains, there will not be enough hours in the day to burn the calories necessary to avoid conversion to fat.

You may choose oatmeal for breakfast or brown rice for dinner. Whole-grain pasta or two slices of sprouted bread are allowed. You are allowed only one serving of whole grains per day, and at no time are you allowed to consume a refined grain (white flour product).

This may be a good time to get to know Quinoa. This is a grain that actually supplies a complete protein.

Rule Three–No trans fatty acids or hydrogenated oils.

Obesity often is caused or supported by the consumption of trans fatty acids. Trans fatty acids are caused by partial hydrogenation of vegetable oils. They are also caused by heat. Any vegetable oil heated above 220 Degrees F can become a trans fatty acid.

Use cold pressed, extra virgin olive oil at room temperature. If you want to sauté something use butter, coconut oil, palm oil or fat rendered from organic bacon. Forget what you have been told about saturated fat. We have been avoiding it for 30 years and look at the trouble people are in with cholesterol and other blood lipids. Remember, saturated fats convert to energy just like a carbohydrate. If one consumes an excessive amount, it too stores as fat. Moderation at all times is important.

Rule Four–Only one fruit or serving of berries or cherries per day. Eat the whole fruit and do not juice it.

Too much fruit can cause unwanted pounds. We forget that the sugar in fruit converts to glucose and fat. The fiber is important and so are the bioflavonoids and enzymes from dark fruits and berries.

I could not count the times I have coached people who are struggling with their weight while consuming large amounts of fruit to avoid fat. This is one of the greatest misconceptions to be thrust on us by the system. They convinced us that fat was making us gain weight. Thirty years of "fat free" dieting has not had an impact on our collective weight as a nation. As a result we have consumed more sugar in every form while avoiding the fat in every form. In the process we have neglected our essential fatty acids. Without our EFAs we do not have optimum metabolism, we are at greater risk for diabetes and cardiovascular diseases.

Studies have shown that consumption of large amounts of fruit juices can contribute to obesity, much the same as soda and sports drinks. The fruit sugar, fructose, is a six-carbon molecule and will produce only half the amount of glucose as table sugar or high fructose corn syrup, which have twelve carbons in their molecule. Fructose has only half the impact on a person's sugar load as commercial sweeteners, but still it contributes to the production of glucose in a body that needs to burn reserves of fat. Also, bear in mind the findings reported earlier about the way fructose processes in the liver similar to alcohol.

Also, many juices are sweetened with concentrations of grape juice or other forms of fructose which correspondingly increases their contribution to the sugar load. Some fruits can be placed in the vegetable category and consumed daily. That would include tomatoes and melons.

Rule Five–Eat only lean servings of meat, poultry and fish. Trim off the fat. Eat only organic or pasture fed, free range meat and poultry. Eat only wild, not farm raised, fish. Also, choose free range or organic eggs.

If you are vegan or vegetarian you may increase your intake of beans and Quinoa to replace the meat. You may also use Edamame or tofu. However, if you choose soy products be cautions that they are not genetically modified. Also, highly processed soy products such as meat mimics and non-fermented soy products are not within the boundaries of this plan.

As we discussed earlier, the rBGH growth hormone used to add weight to cattle and increase dairy production remains in the food products and can have an impact on those who consume them.

In addition to the growth hormones and high-acid grains, pen fed meat also carries the risk of antibiotic residue. Farm raised fish are raised on grains, an unnatural food for fish. Farm raised fish carry more contaminants than wild fish because of their diet and environment.

Grass or pasture-fed cattle have a very different food profile from pen fed animals. The free range meats have only about 10% saturated fat. They will contain the important essential fatty acids such as Omega 3. They also contain CLA, conjugated linoleic acid, part of the essential fatty acid matrix that actually helps release stored fat for conversion to energy. Pasture-fed animals have a pH close to the desired 7.2.

Grain-fattened cattle on the other hand have a much higher acid reading. They have a saturated fat ratio as high as 70%. They have virtually no Omega 3 or CLA. Grazing animals by nature eat grass and other greenery. Feeding them seeds changes everything. The fat from grain fed animals converts to glucose. So people on high-protein diets eating lots of steak might as well eat the grains they are trying to avoid as a carbohydrate.

Rule Six–Have only one or two servings of milk and dairy. Consume only organic milk in moderation. Raw milk and unpasteurized dairy products are preferred if available. Lactose, or milk sugar, is very fattening and it also contributes to inflammation in the body. Skim milk contains just as much lactose as whole milk and is equally fattening.

Choose dairy products that are not pasteurized whenever possible, such as an imported cheese. Pasteurization locks out most of milk's better nutrients, including most of the calcium. Homogenization creates an oily cloud that tends to clog the veins and cause inflammation. Dairy is another clear demonstration of the misconceptions of the past. There is a big demand for reduced fat milk and fat free dairy products. While the fat can convert to glucose, it is not the culprit in dairy foods. The problem with dairy and weight control is milk sugar, lactose.

Lactose is a 12-carbon molecule. It splits in digestion with half, or six carbons converting to glucose. The other six become galactose, an inflammatory factor. This is the substance that can make dairy have a negative impact on sinuses and other inflammatory conditions. In other words, skim milk and whole milk have the same amount of lactose, and in that regard one is as fattening as the other.

Rule Seven–Have no more than one root vegetable per day.

Potatoes, yams, sweet potatoes, beets, carrots and other roots contain large amounts of sugar. One per day is OK. Many diet plans will exclude root vegetables because of their sugar content. I believe that their nutritional value should keep them in the diet with restrictions. Unless the skins are really scuffed, scrub thoroughly and eat the skins, especially potato skins. The skins contain good nutrition, and much of the nutrition is in the first layer of the vegetable right under the skin. This part is lost when the skin is removed. Sometimes the skin is simply not desirable. If that is the case, then certainly discard it.

Within the above guidelines eat according to your hunger. Studies show that four or five small meals per day can increase weight loss. If your body learns that it may not get another meal soon, it goes into a conservative mode and holds on to everything. When your system learns that more food is coming soon, it is more likely to release the fat stores.

At this point I usually see troubled faces and hear comments claiming I have taken away everything and there is nothing left to eat.

Here are a few things you can eat without restriction:

<u>Beans</u> in any form. They help control weight gain, support weight loss and provide a solid balance of protein and carbohydrates.

<u>Cruciferous vegetables</u> are packed with good nutrition and immune boosters. Cabbage, cauliflower, broccoli and others without limit.

<u>Leafy greens</u> including all kinds of lettuce, spinach, kale, collards, Swiss chard, celery and others. Eat salads, but **No Commercial Salad Dressings.** Cold pressed olive or avocado oil and lemon juice or vinegar.

<u>Raw nuts</u> of all kinds. They are full of good fatty acids, protein and immune and metabolism boosters.

<u>Squash and cucumber</u> offer many varieties and flavors. Some can be eaten raw or cooked.

<u>Eggs</u> are recommended. Up to 10 per week. Soft yellows are the healthiest, but they can be prepared any way you like. Eat the whole egg. I would not eat a raw egg unless I knew where it came from and when.

<u>Garlic, onions, shallots, leeks</u> add flavor and are healthy things to eat. Use them generously to enhance other vegetables.

Vegetables do not have to be bland. If you just boil them and put them on a plate they are bland. Add some butter or olive oil and cook them with herbs and spices. Garlic and onion make everything special.

Do not focus on what you cannot have. Eat all you want as often as you want within the guidelines. Explore a world of flavors and new experiences.

Final Thoughts

You did not get up one morning and decide to make your body something that you are not comfortable in? Actually, it does not much matter how it happened or why. If you are not happy with your body and your energy level, it is within your powers to make changes. And you can begin right now. No special preparation or equipment are needed. It is all inside you and all you have to do is reset your mind and your heart's intentions. I have tried to show how our political system has become an enemy to health and wellbeing. You do not have to be a victim of your life, your government, your weaknesses or anything else. You are only a victim of your own choosing because the power of change is within you. You can do it, and you do not need a magic potion or a skinny coach to do it. You got in the condition you are in from bad choices. All you have to do is make better choices and stick to them.

The first step in believing is to believe in yourself. I often say that it is easy to believe in God, but it can be hard to believe in yourself. We must believe that God made us with as much love and care as anything else in this Universe. We often do not feel worthy and expect less than the best in our lives. But, if we believe in God we must also believe that He does not create flaws. We are created equal to anything else and if we do not feel equal it is from our own thinking that we feel inferior. God did not put us in a body that is supposed to make us feel anything but beautiful. He did not prepare us for a life that is anything but vital and valuable. We must have faith in God's creation that bears our name. He has given us each a message and blessings to share with the world. If we do not remain open to being what God intended for us, the world is incomplete and we are missing the joy that is ours. Have the courage to make your own decisions. Take responsibility for your health and wellbeing. Trust God and your own body to lead you to the joy and fulfillment that comes only from being the you that you were intended to be. Nothing else is reality, and nothing else will ever make you happy and comfortable with yourself.

TOMORROW...

In my next book I plan to write extensively about microbes. Were they the beginning of life on Earth, or did they exist before the formation of Earth? Were they formed by the Creator and encoded with the DNA template that would lead to complex life forms? These are common questions circulating among scientists involved in microbiology, Quantum physics and cosmology today. There are many questions and many answers in our immediate future. For the present we should all become familiar with the term, microbiome.

Microbiome is the word that has evolved as acceptable for reference to the one hundred or so groups of bacteria that make up our symbiotic bacteria. They are specialized microbes also known as phyla. Four families dominate our phyla: actiobacteria, bacteroidetes, firmicutes and proteobacteria. These friendly little micro-organisms take care of digestion, control elimination and other normal body functions. Perhaps most important, they are our immune system, and in that function are being considered as important as any single organ of the body. Science is realizing that all life forms depend on micro-organisms to sustain life as we know it. That includes the little bacteria that release nitrogen in the soil to sustain the might oaks, or the gut flora that take care of our digestion, even the production of some vitamins that are not in our diet.

At this point sparse and sometimes primitive experimentation has concluded that there is a direct relationship between a lack of some phyla and disease conditions, including obesity. However, while the connection is irrefutable it is not clear if the lack of certain phyla is a symptom of the condition or the actual cause. It is shown conclusively that restoration of these bacteria can remove the symptoms of the condition. In some minds that is a cure.

I did not include this information in this book as a contributory factor in obesity because the data is not sufficiently conclusive at this time. It is something to watch closely in the future and perhaps we will see a shift in the basic paradigm of medicine from a military, "kill the enemy" approach to one that is more nurturing. In the future we may cure diseases not by trying to kill germs, but by introducing friendly bacteria to the body ecology that will provide a pathway for the healing.

The Author

Gene Ladd grew up in the mountains of Western North Carolina near Asheville where he experienced his first vision quest when he was only ten years old. His earliest memories are hiking the Blue Ridge and Swannanoa Mountains with his Cherokee grandfather wildcrafting herbs. "Diggin' the sang" as it was called in the 1930s. His journey includes a career in radio and TV in New York City and a series of businesses, one of which was a health food store. Now in his late seventies he has evolved into a respected Natural Health Consultant and Spiritual Coach. His healing services, workshops, or private consultations have been called life changing.

"My mission is empowerment, helping people find the energy within for healing and guidance in life."